D1448805

Managing Your Allergies

David Hazard

HARVEST HOUSE PUBLISHERS
Eugene, Oregon 97402

Cover by Left Coast Design, Portland, Oregon

Advisory

Readers are advised to consult with their physician or other medical practitioner before implementing the suggestions that follow.

This book is not intended to take the place of sound medical advice or to treat specific maladies. Neither the author nor the publisher assumes any liability for possible adverse consequences as a result of the information contained herein.

MANAGING YOUR ALLERGIES
Copyright © 2002 by David Hazard
Published by Harvest House Publishers
Eugene, Oregon 97402

ISBN 0-7369-0483-2

Printed in the United States of America.

02 03 04 05 06 07 08 09 / BP-CF/ 10 9 8 7 6 5 4 3 2 1

Contents

Healthy Body, Healthy Soul

People of faith and wisdom have known for ages that our physical body and our inner being are amazingly interconnected. In the Bible, the psalmist wrote about this intricate weaving together of body, mind, and spirit many centuries ago when he observed with reverent awe that we are "fearfully and wonderfully made."

Today, science is rediscovering this important fact: If one aspect of our being is weak or sick, eventually our whole being will be affected. Fortunately, we're learning the opposite is true, as well: When we create health in any single aspect of our being, we benefit our whole person. And the best way to care for ourselves is to take a whole-person approach to curing ailments—an approach that balances physical, mental, and spiritual strategies to restore health and well-being.

Managing Your Allergies offers this approach by addressing the needs of the whole person. It recommends natural healthcare remedies that power up your immunity, equipping your whole being to battle allergens. And it also offers other strategies that help you control or relieve specific allergy symptoms that can make life miserable.

All the strategies offered here are simple and natural. Some have been discovered only recently, while others have been used for centuries by men and women troubled by the same distresses you experience.

This book is not offered as a substitute for support you may need from healthcare professionals, such as physicians or allergists. Neither is it intended to replace a psychological counselor or member of the clergy in cases where personal and spiritual counseling may benefit you.

Ultimately, though, many studies show that we are most likely to find the route back to good overall health—and even achieve healing—when we take personal responsibility for our own health and well-being.

You are the single most important factor in determining your overall personal wellness. And the actions you take on your own behalf—your commitment to selfcare—will determine how quickly you take back your life from the allergies that are limiting your health and quality of living.

In these pages you'll find a wide range of selfcare techniques, including:

- **Mental and spiritual strategies that will relieve inner conflicts that produce stress and depress immunity, boosting your immune system's power to fight allergens.**

- **A simple plan for discovering and eliminating foods that trigger allergic reactions...along with information to help you create your "allergy-beating" diet plan.**

- **The latest information about natural supplements—herbs, minerals, and vitamins—that build core immunity and alleviate symptoms.**

- **Strategies that will give your physical body a "whole-body boost" that restores your energy and increases your strength, helping you to overcome those allergies!**

Because our allergy profiles, and the symptoms they cause, are unique to each one of us, this book doesn't offer a one-size-fits-all program. But it does offer you a variety of natural strategies, old and new. By trying them you will soon learn which ones benefit you the most and eventually tailor a natural allergy relief battle-plan that works for you.

As you find the remedies that work for you, may you experience freedom from your allergies, new vitality, and a return to top health...in *body and soul!*

David Hazard
Founder of The New Nature Institute

1

Create a Shield of Defense

Do any of these situations sound familiar?

You're visiting friends in their home, and just starting to have a great time…and then your eyes start to burn and your airways tighten. Another good time ends prematurely as you are forced to escape whatever allergens are making you miserable.

You've looked forward to this celebration a long time—this chance to be with friends on a great occasion. Then, after just a few bites of dinner, you feel a reaction coming on. Something in the food—maybe an additive, maybe some food ingredient—is beginning to wreak havoc inside you. In a few minutes you're going to be seriously ill….

The gray weeks of early spring are coming to an end. Outside, the moist scent of the earth is sweet, and the trees start to bud and young leaves open…and pollens explode into the air. Once again you have to cage yourself indoors with all the windows closed if you want to breathe. So much for enjoying the returning light and fresh air….

Those of us who suffer with allergies know how life-limiting they can be. While other people can relax and enjoy life, we have to stay on our guard almost all the time.

Whether it's a serious concern about…*insect bites…certain foods or food additives…pet dander…pollens and air quality…the scent of perfume*…we can't just enjoy life as it comes. We have to be on constant guard and take special precautions much of the time. We have memorized our lines as though they were part of our life's script.

- "Does this have dairy in it?"

- "Do your dogs stay in the house?"

- "Is there an outside deck where we can visit?"

- "Will some adult on this hike be willing to take responsibility for my child's bee-sting kit?"

- "Has this skin lotion been tested to be sure it's non-allergenic?"

What makes it even more difficult is that other people often just don't get it. How often have we heard

- "Oh yeah. I guess we knew about your allergy to dairy products—but we didn't think the little bit we used in this recipe would make you *that* sick."

- "We kind of thought you were kidding when you said that pet dander would make your eyes swell and burn. Our pets are in the house all the time, and it never bothers *us.*"

- "Gee, I didn't think it would make your sinuses close *entirely* and give you *that* bad a headache."

When you live with allergies, life can be very difficult, can't it? You feel like you have to live on your guard all the time.

Wanted: A Protective Shield

Wouldn't it be great to have some kind of protective barrier between us and all those allergens lurking out there? To have an invisible "shield of defense"?

Actually, you *do* have a protective shield like that. It's called your immune system. Unfortunately, for millions of allergy sufferers, our defense system has a weakness in it at some point. Certain substances in the environment—whether airborne, or in our food, or delivered in an insect bite—can scramble our immune defenses. As a result, instead of functioning in a normal, healthy way, our bodies go haywire.

Scientifically speaking, we know what happens in an allergy attack: The microscopic particles of some outside substance sweep into our personal world. They land on our outsides—on our skin, on our hair, or in our eyes—or we take them into our lungs or digestive tract. This happens all the time, with countless plants, mineral, and animal micro-particles swirling through our environment—but something about *this particular* substance triggers an alarm in our body that shouts, *"Enemy invader!"* Our immune system quickly mounts a counterattack and struggles to send out its own reinforcements—known as *antigens*—to defend the site of "invasion" against this enemy. But our body can't figure out how to handle this particular invader. The terrible symptoms we suffer are the painful signs of the personal "allergy war" our body is waging.

Knowing that this is how the war starts, medical science has also come up with a standard, prescribed way to help our body fight it. We're tested, to pinpoint the allergens that trigger this hyperactive response in our body. Then, injections containing minute amounts of our allergens are injected into our bloodstream. The point is to "desensitize" us over time by giving our body a chance to deal with small, manageable invasions of the enemy substance. Hopefully, our body will then figure out the right formulation of antigens to overcome the invader…*without* putting us through the miseries of the battle.

What happens in the meantime, though—while our body is trying to figure out a healthy battle strategy? Medical science has more useful strategies.

If the reaction gets out of control, we can take certain prescription drugs to get us through a severe attack. If our bronchial passages and lungs are closing up, we can inhale certain medications which will open them up again and allow us to breathe. If our body is overreacting in other ways—such as a reaction to poison ivy that runs wild over our skin, making life a nightmare of itching—we may be given steroids to shut down our immune response.

Unfortunately, these drugs have limitations and side effects. Bronchial dilators, used a lot and over time, can affect our heart and blood-pressure…and they can also lose their effectiveness.

Because drugs like steroids are so strong and have very negative effects if we use them over a long time, they form a kind of "final line of defense." We don't want to rely on them too long or in excess, because they can cause organ damage and even trigger mood swings into depression.

Become the Captain of Your Own Healthcare Team

The strategies medical science offers *are* important to allergy sufferers, for sure. In a way, they're modern miracles. Not even 100 years ago, the rate of childhood deaths due to asthma was tragically astronomical. If you had handed an inhalant medication to a nineteenth-century mother whose child was dying of asthmatic asphyxiation, she would have thought you were an angel of mercy sent from heaven.

Medical science *has* worked many wonders—and preventing deaths and relieving other life-limiting miseries caused by allergies rank among those nearly-miraculous accomplishments.

We can take advantage of the best the medical world has to offer…especially when we're in a crisis or in absolute misery.

HAVE YOU CONSULTED WITH AN ALLERGIST?

∿

If you suspect that you have allergies and you're putting off a visit to an allergist—don't delay any longer. Make an appointment to see one as soon as possible.

Allergies can affect you in ways that go far beyond the immediate reactions and symptoms you experience. Like any major health condition, allergies have a kind of shock-wave effect on our whole being. They put stress on our physical body, and many of these stresses can be very damaging—weakening our heart, restricting our breathing, and wearing down immune function so we're susceptible to more (and more serious) illnesses. In time, too, the stress of battling with allergies can limit the way we think about life…and cramp our approach to living.

Find a good allergist, and make them part of your personal healthcare team.

But even healthcare professionals would agree that the best care begins when you become the "captain" of your personal healthcare team. Since *your* health and well-being is at stake, shouldn't you be the one who takes the lead in learning how to maintain it?

When we assume ultimate responsibility for our own well-being, we start to make big strides toward recovering health and well-being.

Many of us could begin by refusing to "make room" for poor health conditions we allow ourselves to suffer with. Many of us have learned to "put up with" allergies without taking into account how much they limit us or the collateral effects they have on our health.

By taking responsibility for our health, we stop abandoning our own cause. We stop allowing allergies to determine how, and how well, we'll live. We stop being passive and stop believing that someone else—a doctor or a specialist—is the one who should "fix" us. When we become energized on our own behalf, scientific studies show, we're far more likely to experience a restoration of the good health we once enjoyed.

Second, who but *you* can tell how well a treatment is working? When you take responsibility for your own selfcare, it becomes your job to notice what goes on in your body—and not just when allergens are troubling you, but also when a new kind of treatment is actually having a positive effect. The focus on getting to a resolution keeps you moving forward, trying new strategies, paying attention to your body and its reactions, and keeping your eyes on the goal of better health.

Taking charge of your own selfcare doesn't guarantee that you'll find a magic cure or experience *perfect* health. But it definitely does mean you'll get the best all-around care you can find. *And* it means you're more likely to find the treatments that work best for you—allowing you to manage your allergy symptoms in the best way possible and experience life beyond the limits you're living with right now.

The "Whole-Person" Approach to Health and Wellness

Unfortunately, allergies cause more damage than just the physical reaction you so clearly experience.

As we've seen, allergies put a drain on our immune system. When this important function of the body is on overload, stress is placed on *our whole* physical being—including our circulatory, respiratory, endocrine, and nervous systems. When we're under an allergy attack, every system responsible for good overall health is gradually worn down. We're more susceptible to colds and viruses, and we can be open to more serious infections and illnesses. And we've only touched on the fact that allergies can negatively affect our *inner being*, too. We may live inside mental boxes of worry, fear, and even depression. We can be held back from pursuing our spiritual goals and values.

Since a major health condition such as an allergy affects our whole being, it makes great sense to take a *whole-person* approach in treating it.

In keeping with a current trend in healthcare today, this book offers a whole-person approach to managing allergies and relieving the distressing symptoms they cause. The benefits of taking a whole-person approach to allergy relief include these:

- We address the needs of our whole being—body, mind, and spirit. This means we're taking the surest possible route back to great overall health.

- We don't just ease symptoms—we resolve underlying stressors that erode our health and open us up to attacks. By using physical, mental, and spiritual strategies to restore balance throughout our whole being, we restore our body's natural, God-given ability to defend and heal itself.

- We'll have knowledge of the best whole-body tonics and treatments that natural medicine offers—including herbs, minerals, and vitamins that are known to boost immunity, cleanse the body of foreign invaders, and contribute to ultimate allergy relief. This means we have options besides pharmaceutical drugs. And if pharmaceuticals are causing unpleasant side effects, we may be able to discontinue using them.

- Finally…we can choose from a whole range of natural self-care strategies. This offers us many options for dealing with allergies, so we can find the ones that work best for our individual lifestyles.

Because we were created by God with a body, mind, and spirit—and because all three aspects of our being can become involved when our health is threatened—it only makes sense to use a whole-person approach to restoring wellness naturally.

How This Book Can Benefit You

Each of the following chapters offers solid, up-to-date information about natural selfcare techniques that can help you find relief from your allergies. You will find a wide range of strategies to assist you in building a better "shield of defense"—a stronger immune system. You'll learn:

- How to create a personal allergy-beating diet and eating plan.

- The latest word on natural supplements—which herbs, minerals, and vitamins strengthen immunity, and which ones relieve specific allergy symptoms.

- Strategies to increase physical strength, stamina, and energy—in place of that run-down, wiped-out feeling allergies leave you with.

- Simple techniques to resolve the mental stressors that wear down immunity.

- Spirit-lifting practices—most of them used for centuries—that relieve deep-level stress, allowing your immune powers to increase.

You'll also find more important information in "sidebar" articles throughout to help you fine-tune your personal allergy-resistance plan.

START YOUR OWN
"ENVIRONMENTAL PROTECTION AGENCY"

~

The E.P.A. is a government agency that helps keep our environment safe and clean. Every one of us allergy sufferers needs to become our own personal Environmental Protection Agency—creating the cleanest, healthiest home environment possible.

Here are some of the most important things you can do to make your home a healthy haven where your immune system is not being taxed, but well supported:

1. *Buy an electro-static filter to use on your home heating and air condition system.* Normal air filters, made of nylon mesh, do not do the best job of filtering and cleaning the air in your home. Dust and allergens just keep recirculating. An electro-static filter sifts out the tiniest airborne particles, providing cleaner air to breathe. If you live in a home that has central or baseboard heat, you can purchase an electronic air filter to cleanse the air.

2. *Watch the humidity.* If the air in your house gets too dry—because you're in a dry climate or because the heat is on—the mucous membranes in your nose and throat will dry out and be unable to do their job. *Humidify* when necessary to keep the air compatible with good breathing.

   Likewise, some climates and certain times of the year bring more moisture in the air. Moist, dark basements and closets, and damp upholstery, make excellent environments for molds and mildews. When their spores hit the air, your immune system has to work overtime every minute you're in your own home. Use *dehumidifiers* when necessary.

3. *Keep carpeting and draperies to a minimum.* If you have wall-to-wall carpets, keep them vacuumed. If you can use throw rugs instead, buy the kind that can be washed or shaken out easily.

4. *When choosing a pet, choose wisely.* The best pets for allergy sufferers are those that can live inside glass, outdoors, or at most, in one room of your house. Pet dander is one of the most powerful allergens on earth.

Remember: A healthy home environment is one that gives your whole being a place to relax and rebuild—without the stress of fighting allergens. With a bit of worthwhile effort, you can turn your home into the "protected" space you really need.

Find Natural Allergy Relief—Today

Allergies have limited you long enough. You *can* do something about it.

You can set out in a new direction today. You'll find, throughout this book, a range of natural allergy-relief strategies for building a personalized selfcare plan.

What you need to know are the right strategies—the ones that work for you. And you can start to learn about them right now....

2

An Allergy-Beating Diet

*I*n the whole-person approach to allergy relief, one of the most important—even foundational—changes you can make is to eat an allergy-beating diet. Along with building a healthy home environment, it's one of the most important things you can do for your health, *period*. Diet is vitally important to allergy sufferers because what you eat—and what you don't eat—is critical in building and maintaining strong immune function *and* relieving those irritating allergy symptoms.

Perhaps you've thought that diet is important only for those who are suffering specifically from "food allergies." But that's not so.

For one thing, when you have any allergy, your immune system is under assault. When this important system of your body, which requires great energy to run, is working extra-hard, there is a drain on every other system, including your digestive and endocrine systems. Your body is having a sympathetic response—meaning that all its other systems are working hard to help and to compensate for your battling immune system. Hormones and enzymes are being alternately suppressed...then taxed. This means you're putting out a lot of energy just to maintain a normal level of activity.

Is it any wonder that when you're under fire from allergies you feel exhausted? And there's another factor.

Your immune system is largely located in your lower intestinal tract. It's from here that "allergy-detectors" are sent out to search the body for foreign invaders. When you are under assault by allergens you may feel them most acutely in another part of your body—say, in your itching, runny eyes...or in your swollen, pressured sinuses...or runny, tingling nose...or the itchy, burning rash on your skin...or in your tight airways and laboring lungs. But you are

17

also being assaulted deep down inside…down in your gut, where your immune system is working to send out more and more and more fighters to rush to the site of the attack and to scour the bloodstream for invaders. This means your digestive system is under assault, too.

This is why, in the midst of a battle with allergies, the thought of eating even your favorite foods doesn't seem really appealing… and why sometimes you can feel a little nauseous.

Finally, attention to diet is important for allergy sufferers because we can have *dominant allergies*—that is, allergies that are obvious because their symptoms are pronounced (the itching, sneezing, headaches, and wheezing). But we can also have allergies that have lesser symptoms, or symptoms we mistake for something else. These can be referred to as *sub-dominant*, or "minor" allergies. Often we can have a minor affliction of a food allergy (for example) and not be all that aware of it.

Jerry had been allergic to several pollens and tree saps as a child. If he touched certain plants or trees, his skin erupted with tiny blisters that were filled with clear lymphatic fluid and that itched horribly. He learned to control the reactions and was sure he'd mastered his allergy problems. For the next 25 years, he experienced flare-ups only occasionally, when he worked outdoors in heavy brush. He remained so focused on *this* allergy, though, that he hardly paid attention to the poor digestion and bloating he began to experience at around age 40. Jerry chalked these symptoms up to "approaching middle age." But when he experienced minor bleeding during elimination, he investigated further and learned that he was actually having a lesser allergic reaction to wheat.

Some evidence seems to indicate that for some people, allergic reaction *itself* does not necessarily remain constant. We can develop other, milder allergies that don't always show up as strongly as the original allergy. Many times, we can experience milder forms of food allergies—sometimes called "sensitivities"—and not know what we're dealing with.

So…while diet is obviously important to people with food allergies, it's also very important to *every* allergy sufferer.

The main question then, is this: What kind of diet should an allergy sufferer eat? And how can we detect whether or not a certain food we're eating is actually part of our problem, either because we're allergic, or because we have a sensitivity to it?

The two important strategies in this chapter will help you handle both issues. The first will help you discover reactions to foods you're eating. The second will provide you with important information about the kind of diet that builds immunity and helps overcome allergies.

Strategies for Creating Your Allergy-Beating Diet

Strategy #1: Use an "Elimination Diet"

Most of us are surprisingly unaware of the effects our eating has on us. Sure, we're well aware of obvious things, like heartburn and indigestion. Or a sugar-rush, followed by a crash. But sometimes the foods we eat have an effect that creeps up on us over time…and shows up in minor symptoms we can easily overlook for awhile.

Becoming more mindful of what we eat and how it affects us is important in managing our overall health *and* in relieving allergy suffering. To eat mindfully means noticing what we eat and its effects, as well as focusing our total diet so that we're eating for health and well-being.

This first strategy will help you:

- *Understand* your greater eating patterns (which is important for a number of general health reasons).

- *Recognize* even subtle changes in your body that occur when you have a food allergy, or when allergies are causing you to have a sensitivity to a certain food…so you know what to eliminate from your diet.

- *Detect* the foods that give you a solid, overall boost, allowing you to feel healthy, vital…and great!

If you are working with a healthcare professional, he or she may have other specific guidelines to help you with an elimination diet, but what follows are the most important basics.

Do This

1. **Choose a target time-period.** For 14 days (minimum) focus in on how a certain food group or food affects you.

2. **Choose a target food, or food group.** It's possible you have one or more "suspects" in mind already. Or maybe not. Dairy, wheat-products, red meats—these are the easier allergies or sensitivities to detect. You may want to pick one of these food groups to start with.

3. **Plan how you will eliminate it from your diet.** To do a successful elimination diet, you need an alternate plan. You need to know what you'll *replace* a certain food group or food with in your diet. If you don't, you're likely to give in during the 14-day elimination period and go back to eating the food you're trying to cut out…which means you're likely to miss recognizing what effect it has on you.

4. **Keep a "Better Choice" Notebook.** Keep a notebook at hand. Devote a page to each day. Divide each page in half. On the top half, write:

   I Am Not Eating: (List the food or food group you're eliminating.)

   Instead I Am Eating: (List the replacements.)

Because our eating habits—including *what* we eat—are deeply ingrained, writing down the food you're eliminating each day reinforces the elimination pattern you're trying to establish. And writing down the replacement food is a good way to remind yourself you're not being punished with deprivation.

Now, on the bottom half of each page, write:

   Slips: (Keep things honest—and if you do slip up, no problem; but you'll need to begin the elimination period again.)

   I Felt: (Record any reactions you experienced— including physical reactions and significant mood changes, even those not associated with external events.)

I See: (Capture any daily observations about the interplay between food and your reactions.)

Create 14 of these pages, and on the fifteenth page, write:

Changes: (Note significant changes you noted in your digestion, respiration, moods, sleep habits, or anything else of significance during this elimination period.)

Note: *Remember to eliminate only one food group or food at a time. Some foods will be harder to eliminate—such as processed wheat, which is omnipresent in so many foods. If you suspect that you're allergic or sensitive to a certain food group or food, you should try a second round of elimination until you're certain. Anyone who suffers from cyclical conditions—including PMS or chronic illnesses that regularly flare up—is likely to need the help of an allergist to ultimately determine whether what they're experiencing is related to their diet.*

Food Additives

Food additives can be a potent source of allergic reactions—and they're present in many of our processed foods.

You may need the help of a doctor and further allergy testing to determine whether or not you're allergic to an additive.

Until then, you should at least acquaint yourself with the additives in the foods you have sitting on your shelves at home right now. Go ahead—pull some cans and packages from the pantry, and read the labels.

You'll be amazed to find, for instance, how many foods contain Monosodium Glutamate (MSG)...which is sometimes hidden in our foods under the sneaky term, "natural flavors." You'll also be surprised by the amount of food dyes, which can cause a variety of unpleasant reactions.

If you're serious about an elimination diet, you're smart to take the time and care to determine if additives are causing your allergic reactions.

Strategy #2: Eat an Allergy-Beating Diet

There is no one diet plan that can single-handedly eliminate allergies. If someone tells you that you can eat certain foods and "cure" your allergies…exercise caution! There is no one miracle food, and no combination of foods you can eat will "heal" your allergies.

There is, however, an eating plan that *is* allergy-beating because it

- dramatically increases immune function
- delivers the maximum number of phytochemicals (natural plant medicines), which protect us from toxins in our environment—including both pollution and allergens
- does not stress our bodies by draining hormones and energy for digestion
- helps produce healthy red blood cells to carry oxygen throughout the body and fight foreign invaders

What follows is not some kind of exotic diet. Rather, it's good, sound nutritional advice that will give you the health benefits just described. This diet includes these three features:

1. It offers important recommendations for eating the major food categories—carbohydrates, proteins, and fats—in a given ratio to each other. This balances your metabolism, minimizes stress on your digestive system, and gives you maximum energy.

2. It points you to specific foods within each major category that are known to promote healthy digestion and strong immune function.

3. It doesn't limit you in your eating choices the way many diet plans do. Instead it offers variety so you can pick and choose your own favorites—which makes it more likely you'll stick with it for a long time!

Here, then, is an allergy-beating diet plan you can try for yourself. It begins with our main calorie source.

Good Carbohydrates

A healthy diet is high in complex carbohydrates such as fruits and vegetables. It's slightly lower in proteins, and also low in fats. (We'll get to those.) The complex carbohydrates are primarily found in fruits and vegetables. You will want to add more fruits and vegetables to your diet and greatly reduce your intake of simple carbohydrates, such as pastas and breads.

This rule—more fruits and vegetables, less pasta and bread—is important for overall healthy eating in general. Why? Because simple carbohydrates stimulate insulin production. Early in life, insulin helps the cells assimilate food nutrients for energy and cell reproduction. But in time, our cells become insulin-resistant. They turn away food-energy. So the food energy we used to use to run all systems of the body...now gets stored as fat.

If you're eating to build immune resistance, then getting your carbohydrates from plant sources is very important. That's because plants are rich in phytochemicals (there are thousands of them) as well as vitamins, minerals, and fiber—all immune-boosting. Don't look at these as "just foods"—they're plant medicines that promote total health!

- They are filled with natural antioxidants, which cleanse the blood of free radicals.

- They stimulate the production of the immune system's T-cells and microphage cells.

- They protect healthy cells and organs from environmental toxins.

Fruits. Consider the benefits you can receive by eating more:

- **Apples.** Every type of apple you might enjoy is high in the super-antioxidant quercetin. Apples are also high in fiber, which cleanses the colon. If apples aren't your thing, and you'd prefer another fruit you can buy year-round with similar benefits, go for *pears.*

- **Bananas.** An excellent way to replenish potassium and other important minerals leeched from the body when an allergy attack has stressed you. Also a good source of fiber.

- **Berries.** These little dietary powerhouses are rich in the phytochemicals *lycopene* and *ellagic acid,* both of which help prevent the cell damage allergens often cause. There is also an abundance of antioxidant vitamins in berries—especially blackberries, blueberries, boysenberries, cranberries, raspberries, and strawberries.

- **Citrus.** Some nutritionists recommend reducing the acid in your system, especially when your body is under stress. They recommend keeping your system more pH-basic (which apples and pears will do for you). Other nutritionists recommend that you not eliminate citrus, but instead just go lightly on the **grapefruits, lemons, limes, oranges, tangerines.** Citrus fruits are known to be rich in almost 60 different phytochemicals that boost immunity.

- **Mangoes.** This powerhouse fruit is high in beta-carotene and other carotenoids—even higher than **apricots** and **cantaloupes**, which should also be part of your regular diet.

- **Papayas.** Also rich in betacarotene, papaya is packed with Vitamin C—making it doubly-strong as an immune-booster.

- **Red Grapes.** More often associated with heart-healthy diets, red grapes are high in antioxidants, which cleanse the blood of free radicals. The skin also contains *tartaric acid* (as does the skin of **raisins**) which helps fight diseases of the lower intestines, so they directly protect your immune system.

Grains. Some grains can be a bit hard to digest. Others—particularly wheat—often trigger allergic reactions that can masquerade as indigestion or ulcerative problems. Some grains are as high in protein content as meat, making them a good replacement food if you're serious about trying an elimination diet—and especially if you discover that eating too much meat-protein is hard on you. The most beneficial grains you can eat include:

- **Barley.** This tasty grain is as high in protein as meats are. Because of its nutritional riches, people in some cultures actually live, thrive, work hard, and stay healthy on a diet that is barley-based. It's more versatile than other grains, and can be eaten as a cooked cereal, mixed into soup, or baked into breads. For those who love the chewiness of grain, barley is an excellent choice.

- **Brown Rice.** Whole-grain brown rice is rich in the antioxidant minerals selenium and zinc, and also the bone-building minerals phosphorus and magnesium. When allergies have left you feeling wiped-out, brown rice is a great energy source because it's rich in B-vitamins, and also because it falls in the middle of the glycemic index so it doesn't make blood-sugar levels spike and drop. High in fiber, it also cleanses the system. Some nutritionists consider it a near-perfect complex carb.

- **Oats.** Another heart-healthy choice, oats are a good source of steady energy.

- **Quinoa.** From the Andes, quinoa (*keen*-wah) has the highest protein of any grain (16 percent) and is also a complete protein, with an amino acid profile much like milk. It's rich in iron, for blood-building, and in the B-vitamins and in Vitamin E. Quinoa is very easy to digest, making its energy quickly available to the body. The fact that quinoa places little stress on the digestive system and is a fast re-energizer, plus its general and considerable benefits in a healthy diet, make it a valuable nutritional ally to us all.

Vegetables. Like fruits, vegetables provide us with countless "plant medicines" that boost immunity and promote overall good health. Maybe you've already paid attention to Mom and you always "eat your veggies"…and maybe you haven't. What follows are the best vegetables for improving your total immune function.

- **Asparagus.** Asparagus is high in all the antioxidant vitamins—A, C, E, plus the B-complex vitamins, *and* potassium and zinc…making it a natural and good-tasting "tonic" food for your immune system.

- **Bell Peppers** are rich in antioxidants, thus they give a quick boost to the immune system. While the orange, green, and yellow varieties are high in vitamins like C, the **red bell** peppers hold *three times* as much C and *20 times* as much immune-boosting betacarotene.

- **Carrots.** A rich source of two major antioxidants, Vitamin A and mixed carotenoids, carrots are also high in the B-complex vitamins. You can enjoy raw carrots as a crunchy substitute for snack "munchies."

- **Cruciferous Vegetables—Bok Choy, Broccoli, Cabbage, Cauliflower, Kohlrabi.** All the cruciferous vegetables contain sulforaphane, which helps the body's natural enzymes to fight off toxins and foreign invaders. A potent antioxidant in cruciferous vegetables, lutein protects eyesight and combats respiratory, stomach, and colon distress.

  Note: Cruciferous vegetables are best eaten raw, slightly cooked, or steamed.

- **Dark-Green Leafy Vegetables—Alaria, Arame, Dulse, Hijiki, Kombu, Nori, Sea Palm, Wakame.** If you've never shopped in Asian or specialty grocery stores, you may never have heard of these delicious greens, all of which are rich in immune-boosting phytochemicals. Their flavors range from mild and subtly sweet to spicy and "mustardy" to briny. You'll just have to try them and see which ones you like—or mix them for a great seaweed salad. (Yes, that's what they are.) They can be used in salads and soups, as a side dish, in stir-fries, and as greens on a sandwich.

- **Legumes—especially Aduki, Garbanzo, and Hokaido Beans.** Beans in general are rich in water-soluble fiber, which bonds with waste products in the body for quick elimination, keeping the lower intestines clean. These varieties offer the most health benefits.

  Note: Adding mint to bean dishes can help reduce the discomforts and inconveniences of bloating.

- **Mushrooms—Bolete, Maitake, Morel, Reishi, Shiitake.** These particular mushrooms are important in immune boosters—with Reishis leading the pack. While they are a delicious addition to your diet, you may not want to eat mushrooms in quantity every day. In that case you can still benefit from their therapeutic quality by taking mushroom extract in supplement form.

Your Complex-Carb Goal: To eat for overall good health, make sure that **40 percent of your calories at any given meal come from carbohydrates**—especially from the complex carbs listed above. Eating more vegetables, fruits, and grains has an added benefit, too: It will keep your digestive system working well, and aid in healthy elimination.

R✗

MAKE A "SWEET SWITCH" TO LOCAL HONEY

≈

Many natural healthcare practitioners insist that eating local honey is an excellent way to build resistance to the airborne allergens in your region. For this reason, they recommend that you use honey gathered from *local* apiaries.

Every region has its own pollen combination—a sort of "fingerprint" of the plants growing in that locale. Granted, not all of them flower, but in theory the bees from any given hive will visit enough plants in your area to guarantee that most of their pollens will be represented in the honey the bees produce. By taking in this pollen cocktail with your diet, you may be desensitizing yourself to the ones that trigger allergic response.

Using honey and greatly reducing the sugar in your diet are excellent ideas in any case. Consider making this "sweet switch."

Protein

Certain types of protein are known to promote overall health. Others are known to stress the digestive system, tax our hormonal output, and circulate more acid and toxins throughout the body.

A general word of healthy advice: We need *less animal fat* in our diets. Animal fat—especially red meats—will tend to contain higher amounts of omega-6 fatty acids. This acid is what we know as "bad cholesterol." If our veins and arteries are slowly building up in plaque, our immune system has a harder and harder time combating invaders like allergens. Nutritionists recommend a balance of omega-3 and omega-6 fatty acids—collectively known as essential fatty acids (EFAs).

Many nutritional experts highly recommend a vegan diet, eliminating animal ingredients altogether. We'll discuss the great benefits of plant-based nutrition as we go along. But if you love the taste of meat, don't quit reading. What follows are healthy recommendations about protein choices and their effects on allergy resistance:

- **Chicken.** Many people who are conscientious about their health have switched to eating free-range chicken raised on grain containing DHA. This meat is high in both omega-3s and omega-6s, giving it a healthier balance. If chicken are fed with DHA, you'll find that information on the label.

- **Fish.** In cultures where fish is the main meat source, studies have shown that people are healthier across the board. They experience fewer major diseases (such as cancer and heart disease) and allergies than do people in cultures that consume more red meat. Fish are high in omega-3 fatty acids— the so-called "good cholesterol"—which means they are not clogging your veins and arteries, fighting against your health. And they contain other nutrients important for boosting immunity, including Vitamins B-6, B-12, and folic acid.

  What follows is a list of recommended fish and other seafoods, with the ones most commonly recommended by health and nutritional experts on top:

  >⊃ Anchovies, herring, mackerel, salmon

  >⊃ Albacore tuna, sablefish, sardines

  >⊃ Bluefin tuna, trout

  >⊃ Halibut, swordfish

>○ Freshwater bass, oysters

>○ Sea bass

>○ Pollock, shrimp

>○ Catfish, crabs

>○ Clams, cod, flounder, scallops

- **Turkey.** As with chicken, choose turkey that's been fed grain containing DHA. Turkey is low in the bad fatty acids, making it a better protein choice.

- **Eggs.** Eggs are tricky for people with allergies. The eggs from free-range chickens are your best choice if you don't want to switch to an egg substitute. Since they come from birds raised on the special feed mentioned above, these eggs contain a balance of omega-3 and omega-6 fatty acids.

- **Soy Foods.** Soy foods are an excellent source of plant protein. They provide the immune-boosting benefit of dozens of phytochemicals *and* high protein content. If you're a bit hesitant…you'll be happy to discover there are many delicious soy products including **soy milk, soy cheese, soy burgers, soy mayonnaise, soy sausage, soy bacon, and soy yogurt.**

Soy is also an ingredient in **miso,** a paste used in making flavorful soups and sauces.

Your Protein Goal: The goal of a generally healthy, balanced diet is to have *30 percent* **of your caloric intake coming from protein.** And if you are creating an allergy-beating diet, the goal is to eat more plant than animal proteins.

Fats

We need some fat in our diets in order to make fat-soluble nutrients like vitamins A, D, E, and K do their work. Fat is also needed to trigger the production of many hormones. Contrary to popular opinion, a no-fat diet is *not* a good diet—it's a diet you would go on only if you want to make yourself seriously ill.

Here are some beneficial fat choices:

Butters—nut and seed. If you're eliminating dairy products—have no fear. Better butter choices are available to you.

- **Nut butters**—including **almond butter, cashew butter**, and **natural peanut butter**—are generally a healthy choice.

- **Seed butters**—like **sesame** or **sunflower butter**—are even better choices.

Remember, use any butter sparingly. You only need *a little* fat—not a lot. *Finally,* even though soy was highly recommended above in other food products, *soy butter* is *not* recommended because of its poor nutritional quality.

Culinary Oils—olive, sesame, flax, and hemp. These oils are all high in omega-3 essential fatty acids. Their other importance in health and immune boosting is that they do not become toxic in our system as do other oils that are widely used in our foods.

- **Olive oil** is the oil most often recommended, especially the "extra virgin" variety. It is low in saturated fat, high in important EFAs, and is also known to support liver and gallbladder function.

- **Sesame oil** is the other topflight choice. Readily available in the average grocery store, sesame oil is high in the antioxidant Vitamin E and has as much iron as liver. In addition, it is high in two important amino acids, making it a source of vegetable protein as well.

- **Flax** and **Hemp oils** are also healthy choices…but their taste is a bit strong for some. Since it's all a matter of individual taste, try them and see what you think.

Avoid: Since you want to eliminate fats that become toxic in the body there are three popular oils you'll want to avoid. While **canola oil** has been widely touted as a healthy choice because it doesn't increase cholesterol, it's nevertheless highly refined and very low in omega-3 fatty acids, which means it soon becomes mildly toxic in the body. **Corn oil** is also highly processed and nutritionally valueless. Ignore it. **Soy oil** tastes bitter, is hard to digest, and raises toxicity in the body.

Your Dietary Fat Goal: In a generally healthy diet, about *30 percent* of your total daily caloric intake should come from healthy fats such as those described above.

Drinks

Oddly enough, many people with health conditions including allergies focus on foods to add or eliminate from their diets...and totally overlook what they're drinking.

We'll start with some beverages we can all do without.

You will want to eliminate:

- **Sodas.** Most sodas are unbelievably high in sugar. Check the nutritional info on a can of soda and you'll find that one 12-ounce can contains almost *40 grams of sugar.* That's 10 teaspoons! Eliminating or greatly reducing sugar intake is very important in an allergy-beating diet plan. Yes, you could make the switch to diet drinks...but why not just go totally healthy and learn to enjoy water or natural juices? Sugar not only contributes to body fat and bad dental health, it also contributes to yeast infections in women and is nutritionally valueless.

- **Juices with high fructose corn syrup.** This is another nutritional ingredient that should disappear from every diet. Ever notice how some products say "Juice Drink"—and yet when you read the label, you find out that actual fruit juice is way down on the ingredients list, below water and corn syrup? What you're getting is sugar water with *"up to 10 percent real fruit juice."* (What would happen if you offered the manufacturer "up to" 10 percent of the price they sell these almost-worthless drinks for? Would they like that deal?)

You will want to drink:

- **Green Tea.** It makes a powerful, immune-boosting drink. It's loaded with antioxidants and other important phytochemicals. Drink this healthful beverage hot or cold for a flavorful refresher. Many health-conscious people begin their day with a nice hot cup of green tea.

- **Herbal Teas.** If you love tall, cool drinks—in summer or any time—go with any of the fine flavorful herbal teas available today. Or drink them hot in the cold months. Black teas are fine as well, though you may want to make these a little weaker to cut back on the caffeine.

- **Soy Milk** and **Almond Milk.** Both of these are flavorful, healthy for you, and rich in bioflavonoids (an important supplement you'll read about in the next chapter). Soy milk is as high in protein as cows' milk, but obviously doesn't trigger the allergy symptoms cows' milk does.

3

Nature's Medicines

Some of the natural supplements discussed in this chapter are known to cause negative reactions when taken in combination with prescription medications. Some are also known to cause negative reactions when taken in combination with other supplements.

When a supplement is known to react negatively with a drug or another supplement, these are noted for you, along with other cautionary advice.

When adding natural supplements to your allergy-resistance plan, you should do so in consultation with a healthcare professional. Always notify healthcare professionals before adding natural supplements to your selfcare treatment plan.

Some healthcare experts—the traditionalists and the new naturopaths—argue that we *should* get all our vitamins and important nutrients from our diet. Most traditional doctors say supplementation is unnecessary and largely a waste of money. At most, they recommend a daily multiple vitamin, maybe some extra Vitamin C in the cold, dark months, and maybe an additional mineral for certain conditions—such as extra iron to prevent or resolve anemia.

The fact of the matter is that most of us do not eat the kind of diet that gives us all the nutrients we need. And given the diet of highly-processed food most of us eat—foods so stripped of natural nutrients that they have to be injected back in after processing—it's unlikely we're getting what we need from even a reasonably balanced diet.

Add to that this fact: When we have a health-impairing condition, such as an allergy, we need certain nutrients in far greater quantity than we're likely to get in our regular diet—or even in a relatively healthy diet.

Supplementation *is* both necessary and beneficial.

In this chapter you'll read about herbs, minerals, and vitamins known to have therapeutic value in treating allergies. Additional information in the "sidebar" articles will give you other important information such as how to create topical treatments for skin allergies, how to find out if the supplements you're taking are worth the money, how to know which herbal remedies being sold today are actually harmful, and even how to take supplements safely, wisely, and for the greatest benefit.

What follows are the natural remedies most often used to treat allergies. Make sure to note details about their use, and especially the cautions that might apply to you.

A Natural Apothecary
for Allergy Relief

The Herb Shelf

Nature offers us many herbs that are therapeutically beneficial for allergy relief.

Some of them can be used to ease specific symptoms such as nasal or chest congestion, sinus headaches, rashes, and itching. Others are potent supporters of overall immunity. Some are even considered "super tonics"—called *adaptogens*—because they're known to support the functioning of several major systems of the body at once, including the immune, digestive, respiratory, endocrine, and circulatory systems.

You should approach the therapeutic use of an herb as you would approach the taking of a pharmaceutical drug—that is, with care and with respect for its potency.

Finally, since the phytochemicals in herbs *are* natural medicine, your liver and kidneys will need extra help in processing these substances. Drink between four and eight, eight-ounce glasses of water a day to help flush these organs.

- **Aloe Vera.** Derived from the leaves of the aloe plant, the extract, aloe vera, has been used successfully by gastroenterologists and practitioners of natural medicine alike. It's used to relieve serious digestive-tract distress caused by food allergies. It's also a natural laxative, and its compounds promote the healing of inflammation when the intestinal lining has experienced severe irritation and damage.

  Caution: Used internally, aloe vera can cause severe cramping. For this reason it is not recommended for internal use during pregnancy.

- **Amalaki (Indian Gooseberry).** The extract of this Asian fruit is highly regarded in oriental medicines as an adaptogen—a "super tonic." Because it's known to stimulate the production of healthy red blood cells, it's also recommended by many practitioners of natural medicine for building immune resistance.

- **Astragalus** is a Chinese herb known as an immune-boosting tonic. It's even more effective in stimulating immune response when used in combination with Siberian Ginseng. (See below.) Astragalus is also a good way to re-energize yourself naturally, without side effects, when allergies have worn you down and left you feeling fatigued.

- **Bloodroot** is a blood purifier that comes to us through Native American herbal knowledge. It is used to reduce all symptoms of allergic reaction, and also as a nasal decongestant during cold and flu season. Dried forms are available, but the extract, used in a tea, is more potent and more likely to offer the anti-allergy benefits you need.

- **Burdock (Gobo).** This common weed has been known in folk medicine for centuries as another "purifier." Burdock contains inulin, a compound which stimulates the production of white blood cells, thus increasing the body's overall defenses. It also stimulates liver function, helping with blood purification. *And* it's a mild diuretic, once again helping to detoxify the body. It is sometimes sold in fresh root form under its Asian name, Gobo.

"SALVE-ATION" FROM SKIN RASHES

~

Many of the popular, over-the-counter salves that are sold to treat allergy-caused rashes and itching contain cortisone and other synthetic drugs. You may find that cortisone is too strong for your skin, or you may prefer to try gentler, natural remedies that are, nonetheless, effective.

- **Aloe Vera Gel** (not the clear, watery extract recommended above for internal use) is highly effective in soothing and drying poison ivy, poison oak, and poison sumac. *Caution: Aloe Vera Gel should not be taken internally.*

- **Calendula** is an especially effective herbal treatment for healing skin rashes and calming that irritating itch. Make Calendula into a salve, and you have a potent topical treatment.

- **Comfrey** is a potent inhalant for the relief of nasal and respiratory congestions. You can make a salve of it and store some in a small metal or plastic container to carry with you. Inhaling Comfrey aromatics is recommended, as they have a strong medicinal scent you will probably not want to carry around on your skin.

  To make an easy salve, mix 2 or 3 drops of herbal essential oil (or 2 tablespoons of the dried herb) into 2 tablespoons of a non-allergenic skin cream or moisturizer. Or you can mix the herbs into 1 part each beeswax, cocoa butter, and a plant extract like olive oil.

  Use 2 tablespoons of the base vehicle to 2-3 drops of essential oil or 2 tablespoons of the dried herb.

- **Witch Hazel** can still be bought as a rash and itch-soothing lotion in most pharmacies. It's amazing how we forget how good the old-fashioned remedies really are. As recently as 30 years ago, Witch Hazel lotion was widely used to relieve even the worst itching caused by allergic reactions. *It still works great.* Apply this clear liquid liberally on your tormenting skin rashes with a cotton ball and experience its healing, soothing benefits.

- **Feverfew** comes from the aster family, and has long been known as something of a wonder drug, curing both headaches and "melancholy." When allergies are making your sinuses scream with pain, this may be an herb you should turn to. Its main active ingredient is parthenolide, and is most effective when taken on a regular basis rather than the moment a headache strikes. Feverfew is available in capsules and in raw leaf form.

    Note: *If you are suffering from hayfever symptoms, Feverfew is not a good choice. This herb should also not be used during pregnancy, as it's known to bring on menses. It can also affect blood-clotting, so you should not use it with a blood-thinning medication such as Coumadin or Warfarin, or before or after surgery.*

- **Ginger Root.** Many people carry gingersnap cookies with them when they travel to ease motion sickness. Ginger Root has more potent medicinal uses, due to the healing properties of its most active ingredient, gingerol. In fact, Ginger Root has been used for centuries to help ease stomach distresses of every kind. Use it if food allergies have triggered nausea or cramping.

    You will want to use the fresh root, grated into a tea ball, to make a flavorful, pain-relieving tea.

- **Goldenseal** is wonderful for drying up a runny nose, post-nasal drip, and excess mucus in the throat. Goldenseal is available in dried form in capsules, though the extract is generally considered to be more potent and useful in treating allergy symptoms.

- **Licorice Root.** This herb stimulates your whole system, causing your body to expel excess mucus. For that reason it's often used to relieve colds, allergies, and sinus infections.

    Licorice Root is available in capsules and in extract. The dried herb also makes a wonderful, flavorful tea.

- **Meadowsweet.** The word "aspirin" comes from Spirea, which is an alternate name for Meadowsweet. The connection? Meadowsweet contains salicylin, which the body converts to salicylic acid, which is the active ingredient in aspirin. But

Meadowsweet delivers a much gentler, safer alternative to aspirin. It may take a few minutes longer for the herb to counter your headache, but it's also less destructive to your stomach lining.

Meadowsweet tea is a common way to ingest this herb, which is available in dried form and in extract.

HOMEOPATHY

～

There are many homeopathic substances that are being used to treat allergic responses with a great deal of success. Maybe you've heard or read about some of them in health magazine articles. But before you're tempted to buy them at your local healthfood store, consider this.

Homeopathy is as exacting a healthcare practice as any. Finding the right substance to help you and getting the dose right requires careful monitoring by someone knowledgeable and experienced.

So, if you want to try homeopathy, seek a practitioner who is trained in homeopathic medicines and protocols to treat your allergies.

If you are wondering how to find a trained homeopath in your area, call The American Institute of Homeopathy at (703) 246-9501.

- **Peppermint.** The menthol in Peppermint breaks up congestion.

  Peppermint tea is a widely-used remedy for allergy symptoms such as nasal or chest congestion. Buying the loose herb is likely to be more effective. When buying teabags, check the date on the package.

- **Reishi (Mushrooms).** These oriental mushrooms have powerful immune properties.

Of all the oriental mushrooms used in healing remedies, Reishis are the ones that have been used for centuries to boost the immune system against allergies.

Reishi is available in powdered form in capsules, and in extract.

- **Rhodiola** is a powerful adaptogen that's just coming into use here in the west, though it's been used elsewhere in the world for centuries as a "super tonic." It acts upon the whole body and increases resistance to physical, emotional, and chemical stressors —including, of course, allergens. (Its other great benefit is that it increases the production of serotonin in the brain, causing a deep calm. Because all your energies aren't being drained from you in nervous tension, you will feel more energized, as well.)

  Rhodiola is available in capsules and tablets, or use the dried-leaf form if you'd prefer it as a fragrant, comforting, healing tea.

- **Siberian Ginseng** is one of the most potent whole-body tonics available. When your body is stressed by allergies, you need a good tonic to rebuild foundational well-being. Though it takes two to three weeks for this herb to work, its supportive effects are strong and lasting. There are several kinds of Siberian Ginseng, and you should make sure that one of its scientific names—*eleuthero* or *E. senticosus*—appears on the label, as many substitutes and impostors are being used in its place. The *authentic* Siberian Ginseng fortifies against long-term stress, and it helps keep blood pressure steady.

  Siberian Ginseng comes in capsules and extract, but if you can find it in root-form you can use it to make a great tonic tea. As mentioned above, combining this herb with Astragalus makes for a potent, natural, allergy-resisting tonic.

- **Tulsi (Holy Basil).** This potent adaptogen comes to us from centuries of use in Indian ayurvedic medicine. It's reputed to increase longevity—but if it didn't have immune-boosting and allergy-relieving benefits, who'd *want* to live longer? Like other adaptogens, it's best to use Tulsi on a long-term basis. Use it throughout the year if allergies are a constant problem.

Or you can begin using tulsi four to six weeks before your particular "allergy season" begins.

Tulsi comes dried, in capsule form.

ARE THE SUPPLEMENTS YOU'RE BUYING ANY GOOD?

Some laboratories have tested natural supplements only to find that the substance named on the jar's label doesn't even exist in some of the capsules. Sometimes the quality and potency of the substance varies widely from one manufacturer's lot to the next.

If you're going to take natural supplements to relieve allergy suffering, you want assurance that they're high in quality and potency. And you want to be sure you're spending your money wisely.

Here are two ways you can check out the supplement manufacturers you're buying from:

- **Dietary Supplement Quality Initiative.** DSQI reviews natural supplements and makes its findings available to the public. Read up on the latest supplement news at their website: www.dsqi.org.

- **ConsumerLab.com.** This website posts the findings of dozens of independent labs that buy supplements off-the-shelf, just like many consumers do, and tests them. They test for purity, the accuracy of information on the label, and consistency. Test results are available free by just logging on.

The Mineral Shelf

Just a few minerals are known to have therapeutic benefit in relieving allergies, but as it happens their role can be very important.

- **Selenium** is an effective antioxidant trace mineral. Combined with Vitamins C and E, or with one of the other powerful antioxidants, it breaks down toxic chemicals and allergens we take in from the environment *and* it combats toxins produced by the body itself.

- **Magnesium and Zinc.** These trace minerals taken in combination have a powerful healing effect. Besides performing such basic functions as stimulating healthy cell formation, when combined they combat colds and allergies. You should keep a supply of magnesium and zinc on hand, especially if your allergies weaken you and make you susceptible to colds. This combination of minerals—especially the zinc—can knock a cold out of you in as little as 24 hours if taken every few hours throughout the day. Few things are more miserable—or more taxing on your whole being—than fighting a cold and allergy symptoms at the same time.

EPHEDRA WARNING

～

Epinephrine is a pharmaceutical drug doctors often use to stimulate respiration when asthma is shutting down a patient's breathing. In that case, epinephrine is normally administered in a clinical setting and under a physician's watchful care. Some have referred to Ephedra—an herbal stimulant—as "natural Epinephrine." But...

Healthcare experts warn against the use of Ephedra. Yes, it does stimulate circulation and respiration. (It's often sold in "quick stop" stores to give long-distance drivers a "buzz" to keep them awake on the highway.) But it hits the heart and respiratory system with a powerful jolt, which of course is where the "rush" comes from. That in itself is dangerous. In addition, its effects on the nervous system seriously deplete the body...and then it wears off, triggering a big let-down.

When it comes to using Ephedra to relieve allergy symptoms...don't! Ephedra can be dangerous. Safer natural stimulants are on the market. And be aware—Ephedra is sometimes sold under the name *Ma Huang.*

The Vitamin Shelf

Vitamins are essential for our basic health—and some are highly important in building the greater immune function we need to combat allergens and re-boost our bodies during and after an attack.

Environmental stressors and dietary deficiencies conspire to keep us from getting the vitamins we need normally. And when we're fighting allergies—seasonally, or throughout the year—we need higher doses of certain important vitamins to fight the allergens that have invaded our bodies *and* to restore overall health and well-being.

As is true with minerals, there are just a few vitamins known to have therapeutic benefit to allergy sufferers, but the boost they give is *great.*

- **Vitamin A.** This is one of the most potent of the antioxidant vitamins, all of which are beneficial in fighting allergies.

  A word about the importance of antioxidants: Antioxidants bond with free radicals in our blood and eliminate them quickly from our bodies, before they can do damage. A free radical is a foreign, toxic substance, absorbed from the environment—such as a pollutant or an allergen—or even a toxin created by our body itself in the normal course of taking on food-energy and giving off wastes. When free radicals build up in the bloodstream—which is what happens when we're attacked by allergens—and our whole system becomes stressed, the radicals attack our blood vessels and damage cells throughout the body *and* further suppress immune function.

  Vitamin A heads the list of antioxidant vitamins you will want to include in building allergy resistance.

  Caution: *Unlike most other vitamins, Vitamin A is not water-soluble, which means it can be stored and build up in the body's fat tissues. High doses, taken in a short period of time, can have a toxic effect. Follow manufacturers' directions carefully.*

- **Vitamin B-Complex.** A wide range of important body functions are affected by this family of vitamins. Unfortunately, the B-vitamins are quickly depleted when we are under physical, mental, or spiritual stress. One of the B-vitamins—B-6 (*Pyridoxene*)—is known for its special ability to empower the immune system. It helps in the production of new and healthy red blood cells and the creation of antibodies which protect against foreign invaders. But it's best to take all of the B-vitamins in combination, because together they have an overall tonic effect on the body *and* they give us a needed energy boost by helping our bodies to use food-fuel efficiently.

- **Vitamin C** is another of the antioxidants. Vitamin C is considered so important in building immune function that it's often taken in doses higher than manufacturers' or the U.S. FDA's recommended dosages for diseases both mild and terrible—from common colds to cancer.

  Certain claims have been made about the health and anti-aging benefits of taking C in extremely high doses—up to 100,000 milligrams per day, or *ten times* the maximum recommended dose. You can experience the therapeutic, immune-boosting value of Vitamin C by taking smaller doses than that—say, two or three times the recommended daily dose.

  Caution: *Higher doses of Vitamin C may cause cramping and diarrhea. Though not toxic, this is obviously not healthy or pleasant. If you experience this distress due to an intake of Vitamin C that is too high for your system to tolerate, reduce the dosage you are taking immediately. Be sure to replenish your electrolytes with an increased intake of fluids, preferably water.*

- **Bioflavonoids** (**Vitamin P**). These water-soluble antioxidants greatly enhance the body's absorption and use of Vitamin C. For this reason, they are often sold in combination with C. Derived from fruit and vegetable sources, bioflavonoids include citrin, flavones, flavonols, hesperidin, quercetin, and rutin—and now, when you see them on a label, you'll recognize these unfamiliar names and know the benefit these substances hold for you. (Read more about quercetin below.)

- **Coenzyme Q-10.** "CoQ-10" is a fat-soluble enzyme often found mixed in with vitamins on the shelves of pharmacies and health food stores. This enzyme is naturally produced in both plant and animal cells, where its primary job is to help cells derive energy from nutrients.

Helping our cells get the most energy from passing nutrients is a great benefit when fighting an allergy attack and the fatigue it causes. For this reason, it's very important in restoring vitality. CoQ-10 is also an antioxidant. It works in combination with Vitamin E to prevent damage caused by free radicals.

Caution: Consult with your physician before taking CoQ-10 if you are taking heart medications, as it may react negatively with some of these pharmaceuticals.

- **Vitamin D.** Recent clinical studies have shown that it's important to maintain our intake of Vitamin D, especially during an allergy attack that causes skin irritation or rashes. This is because the skin is a "sun receptor," and the contact with sunlight and heat is what we don't want when an allergy is triggering histaminic skin irritation and itching. Vitamin D is necessary for overall health and the absorption of food-energy into our cells.

- **Vitamin E.** Yet another important antioxidant. By blocking damaging, foreign substances absorbed from the environment, Vitamin E protects cell membranes and boosts immune function.

  Note: Vitamin E, especially taken in higher doses over a sustained period of time, acts as a blood-thinner. For this reason, you should not use it if you are taking blood-thinning medications such as Coumadin or Warfarin. Women who experience difficult menstruation should consult their physicians before using E in higher doses. You should not use Vitamin E immediately before or after a surgery.

- **Quercetin** is one of the most powerful of the bioflavonoids. Rather than addressing the symptoms, quercetin helps to alleviate the underlying allergic response. It does so by stabilizing the membranes of cells that release histamine…"quieting down" an allergic response at its source.

Aromatherapy: Good Sense...
or Just Good Scents?

~

Aromatherapy has emerged in recent years as a way to treat all kinds of ailments and distresses—including allergies. Essential oils are sold in kiosks and shops everywhere.

Skeptics say it's the breathing *itself* that induces better respiration, better blood oxygenation, and mood elevation. They say the scents themselves do nothing.

But scientific evidence says otherwise. When the aromatic molecules of an essence hit the olfactory sensors in your nose they send messages to the limbic system of the brain. Among other things, the limbic system influences your immune system. Aromas *do* trigger immune response.

Even if breathing properly were "all there is" to aromatherapy—that's actually an excellent reason to try it! Any scent that induces us to breathe deeply makes good sense.

Practitioners, including naturopaths and herbalists, insist that certain essential oils have been shown to benefit specific conditions.

To relieve allergy symptoms you may wish to try these:

eucalyptus

hibiscus

peppermint

To use essential oils: Mix 2 to 3 drops maximum of essential oil in bowl with 1½ quarts of boiling water. Put a towel over your head and lean over the bowl, "tenting" the steam. Inhale through your nose.

Pregnant women should not use the following essential oils: basil, bergamot, cypress, geranium, hyssop, marjoram, melissa, peppermint, sage, thyme, or wintergreen. Check with an aromatherapy expert or a knowledgeable healthcare professional before using *any* essential oils during pregnancy.

Prevent children from coming into direct contact with essential oils.

How to Take Supplements

Just *take* them, right? Not so. You need some knowledge about how to take supplements—important knowledge. A few basic facts will help you.

1. **Buy quality.** Price is not an indicator of quality. Go to websites and organizations that test and rate natural supplements, and check out the manufacturer from whom you're buying. (*See above*: "Are the Supplements You're Buying Any Good?")

2. **Read labels carefully.** Some supplements must be taken with food. Others are more effective if taken in several doses over the course of a day. Many manufacturers will also list drugs and other supplements with which this particular substance will react negatively. This can hardly be emphasized enough: *Read the label.*

3. **Increase your water intake.** It is very important to increase your intake of fluids—preferably water—when taking supplements. This means taking in more than the few sips it requires to get the supplements down.

   Increasing your water intake is important because many supplements make your liver and kidneys work harder, and water will help these vital organs do their work better and keep them functioning in a healthy manner. In some cases, you may be taking doses that are several times greater than the normally recommended daily dose, and so your liver and kidneys most definitely need the added help of more water.

   If you are taking natural supplements regularly, drink a minimum of four eight-ounce glasses of water a day, and build up to eight. Cool water, *not cold,* is best.

4. **When taking herbs, more is *not* better.** Certain supplements such as vitamins and minerals do increase in effectiveness if you increase the daily dosage. It does not work the same way with herbs. Herbs are effective and build up potency over time. Upping the dose is a waste and can cause toxicity in some cases.

5. **Give supplements time to work.** Natural supplements of any kind take time to show their effectiveness. They are not like pharmaceutical drugs, which work quickly. In some cases, it may take two weeks or even a month for a supplement to build up to its therapeutic level.

6. **ALWAYS discuss the supplements you are taking with your physician.** Use supplements to enhance, and never to block or counteract, the effectiveness of any other treatments you are undergoing under a physician's care. The presence of a substance in your blood also needs to be known when considering the results of blood tests.

   Even if your physician is not a believer in using natural supplements for allergy resistance, there's no benefit in keeping secrets from your doctor, and it can be harmful. *Don't do it.*

4

Body-Boosting Excercises

For allergy sufferers, engaging in heavy work, exercise, or play can trigger an allergic reaction of one sort or another. For some, the lungs are affected and breathing gets difficult. For others, heat and perspiration trigger the production of histamines, sinuses swell, or skin gets itchy. Our tendency, then, is to avoid exercise altogether.

This is not a good choice.

Avoiding the challenge and fun of good healthy play and exercise limits us. More than that, life without good exercise and play equals poor overall health, weak muscle tone, and greatly decreased immunity. Practically speaking, heavy work is sometimes unavoidable, and we *need* to be strong for work as well as play.

The Better Choice—Body-Boosting Excercises

Since we were made with physical bodies, we *need* a whole variety of physical activities for overall well-being. For too many of us—adults and children alike—too much of our lives is sedentary. We get little or no physical workout and wonder why we don't feel the greatest. If allergy relief is what we're after, however, we can make a better choice.

What we really need is a health plan that includes the kind of activities that give us a whole-body workout—a workout that boosts immune function, restores overall well-being, and helps us feel our best. Excusing ourselves from things like exercise, hard work, or play is the wrong way to go. Because activity that makes us work and

49

sweat contributes to overall good health, we should assume that we *are* going to work out.

The right way to go is to find the best workout routine for you. A good workout not only strengthens your body, it also

- boosts overall immunity
- increases the production of healthy hormones that fight allergies
- creates greater lung capacity, so our normal breathing is deeper and healthier
- promotes better circulation and oxygenates the blood better

We need to learn how to stay active without triggering allergy symptoms that make us miserable. We also need to find a range of physical workouts—some less strenuous, some more—so that we have choices for both bad and good days, maintaining a goal of staying active all the time.

What follows are simple strategies we can use to build or maintain strong, well-toned bodies on a regular basis. We start with the easiest ones, for those days when allergy symptoms leave you feeling limited, and move up the range to those that give you maximum help in boosting lung capacity, immunity, and overall strength.

Body-Boosting Strategies

Strategy #1: Breathe Deeply

One of the absolute basics of good health is good breathing. Believe it or not, there is a way to breathe that boosts overall wellness and immunity. Unfortunately, few of us adults breathe this way normally.

The kind of breathing we do when we're at rest or moving along at our normal pace is usually fairly shallow. The average adult uses only about one-third of our lungs' capacity. In times of stress or tension our breathing becomes shallower still and drops to as little as *one-quarter* of total capacity. If we're under stress at our job, in a relationship, or because of our health, or when we're depressed, we breathe shallowly much of the time. And who among us *isn't* under stress these days?

Two levels of physical distress result from normal, shallow breathing.

First, waste gases build up in our lungs, blood, body tissue, and cells. We feel achy, fatigued, even lethargic, unaware that these are physiological symptoms of the toxins and acids accumulating in the very fibers of our being. We're depriving our bodies of the oxygen needed at the most basic level of life, for healthy cell reproduction. This weakens our immunity.

Second, lung capacity slowly decreases. The lungs don't "shrink," but their ability to take in oxygen and expel toxic gases does diminish. Again, immune function drops.

To boost immunity and overall well-being, we need to practice deep breathing.

Do This

1. **Notice how you're breathing right now.** Normally, we use only the upper chest muscles to inhale, filling just the top part of our lungs with air. Feel which muscles you are using.

2. **Now use your *diaphragm* to help you inhale.** Your diaphragm is the big muscle below your rib cage. You'll know you're using your diaphragm to breathe when you cause your belly to extend. Your chest will only expand a little. (This is the way babies breathe naturally. Sadly, it's a habit that shallow and stressful breathing trains out of us.)

   Note: Deep breathing is likely to make you light-headed unless you refine your technique. So...

3. **Close your lips. Breathe in slowly through your nose.** To slow your inhalation, try breathing in to the count of *five*. Remember to use your stomach muscles. The point is to slowly fill your lungs to full capacity.

   At the peak of your inhale, do not hold your breath. Instead...

4. **Relax your lips, as if you're blowing out a candle. Exhale through your mouth**…but not too quickly. Try it to the count of *three.* This will insure that you clear your lungs fully and that you'll breathe more deeply than normal.

5. **Repeat the pattern for *two minutes.* Concentrate on your counting.** The goal is to keep up the pattern without becoming light-headed from hyperventilating.

You'll find that a two-minute "workout" is enough to begin with.

STAY HYDRATED

～

Many of us are at least mildly dehydrated because the "treated" air we breathe in our homes, work places, or schools sucks the moisture from our bodies.

Add to that an exercise routine, and you can really dry yourself out. As you breathe harder you'll dry out your mouth, throat, and nasal passages (besides generally losing body fluids by perspiration). *And*…if you work out in a health club or community center, the circulated air in many of those places can be *very* dry, depending on the kind of industrial-strength air conditioning and heating units they use. So…

You need to drink plenty of water before and after exercising. And you especially need to hydrate yourself throughout the day if you use more active routines and workouts.

When you keep yourself well-hydrated, you

- help your mucous membranes—an important part of your immune system—to function properly

- keep your electrolyte levels high, preventing fatigue *and* helping your blood cleanse itself quickly from food- or airborne allergens you've taken in

If you're active, do your body—and your immune system—a favor by building up to eight, eight-ounce glasses of water a day.

Strategy #2: Now That's a Stretch

When you roll out of bed in the morning, what's the first thing you do? Stretch—right? And it feels *great*. You stimulate deep breathing and release stress, triggering that all-important deep-relaxation response. Your muscles contract and express toxins that have accumulated overnight. Joints and tendons get loose, blood-flow increases, and your metabolism wakes up...*all that*, from just a simple stretch.

So imagine what a whole routine of stretching can do for you.

Stretching is one of the workouts you can use anytime, but *especially* on those days when allergy symptoms are at their worst and you really don't think you can push it. In fact, stretching is one the most underrated and beneficial physical regimens you can use to improve physical (and even mental) health.

Start or end your day with a simple stretching regimen. Most of these moves can be done at the office, too. (A few can even be used to de-stress and refresh you while you're stuck in traffic or anytime you feel tense and your breathing gets shallow.)

Do This

1. **Sit in an open space on the floor, or in a chair if you need back support.** If you're sitting on the floor, move your legs until they're comfortably apart, and:

   - Begin by loosening your hips, the back of your thighs, and your buttocks. These are the largest muscle-groups in your body. When you were first born, and if you were active as a kid, these were more flexible. The more you've aged, the less you've stretched and firmed these important muscles. So...

   - Slowly lower your torso toward one knee, then the other. Feel the muscles in your hips, buttocks, and back of the thighs stretch.

   - After you stretch each side out, take a cleansing breath...in slowly through your nose...out in a puff through your mouth. (Continue this after each set of stretches recommended.)

The muscles in this area of your body have been called "the second heart," because when they're made to stretch and pump, they increase overall circulation dramatically. And if you want to work against the aging, stiffening, sagging process, these are important muscle groups to keep limber and toned.

2. **Loosen up your neck.** Never roll your head in a circle to stretch the neck muscles, as it's very easy to damage the delicate vertebrae, disks, and nerves in your neck. Instead

   - Tip your head to the left as if to touch your ear to your shoulder. Feel the tendons and muscles on your right side stretch. Repeat on the right side.

   - From the head-up starting position, tip your head forward and touch chin to chest. Feel the back of your neck relax.

   Keeping your neck loose and free of muscle-knots will prevent these muscles from pinching on the nerves passing through them...which sends "tension" and "pain" signals up through your face and head, resulting in that tired-around-the eyes, or dull-headachy feeling.

3. **Loosen your shoulders.** This continues the process of releasing tight trigger points, expressing lactic acid, and increasing blood flow in the neck, shoulders, and torso.

   - Raise your left shoulder to your ear. Then roll it forward and down. (You may hear "clunks" in your shoulder blade. If they're painless, don't worry.) The goal is to feel the muscles between your shoulder blade and spine stretch and relax. Repeat, using your right shoulder.

4. **Loosen your chest and abdomen.**

- Extend your arms, elbows locked, palms down, and place one hand on the back of the other.

- Slowly raise your arms till they're pointing straight up. As you do, breathe in, and feel your diaphragm fill. Reach for the sky, and feel your chest and abdominal muscles stretch.

- Move your arms a little further back until they're behind your head. Clasp hands. Using your right hand, draw your left arm down to the right…and feel the muscles along your left side stretch. Repeat, using your left hand…and make your right side happy.

You are *remembering to breathe through the stretches, aren't you?*

5. **Loosen your calves and quadriceps.**

- Straighten your left leg and point your toes. Feel your shins stretch. Repeat on the right. Push your left heel out…feeling your calf stretch. Now, the right.

- Grab your left ankle. Slowly draw your leg back behind you…and feel the quads on the front of your legs stretch. (Don't over-extend your knee-joint.) Relax. Repeat for the benefit of your right leg.

You've just completed a full-body stretch. You've released stress and toned muscles. You've increased your lung capacity, oxygenated your blood, stimulated your metabolism…*and* helped boost immunity.

Note: *The rule for stretching is to* **go slowly** *and* **move gently.** *Never force a stretch, or you may harm muscles and tendons. Use your fingers to knead and loosen tight muscles as you go along.*

STRETCH *AND* STRENGTHEN...
IN ONE EXERCISE

~

Many workout regimens give strength training *or* stretching and flexibility. Yoga gives you both.

Yoga is a wonderful exercise regimen that has helped people for some 8000 years. Along with stretching your large-muscle groups, it builds muscle strength in a natural way. You can easily find yoga instruction in classes, books, and videos that offer you the health benefits of a light to moderate workout.

If Eastern philosophies are not your thing, don't worry. Many instructors leave out the metaphysical talk and just offer yoga as an exercise.

Strategy #3: Walk Your Way to Greater Immunity

As with stretching, most people undervalue the benefits of a good walking regimen.

Walking at even a *moderate* pace is a great way to improve respiration, increase physical stamina, and strengthen your overall immunity. Add to your daily walk one of the strategies for better mental or spiritual health and you'll be on your way to a "whole person" workout.

Please note, we're not talking about a saunter, but rather a brisk motion. There are a few things you can do to make your walk most beneficial.

Do This

1. **Choose two or three routes.** Try to pick a short route (10-minute walk), a mid-range route (20-minute walk), and a long course (30 minutes or more). This will give you changes of scenery and options to choose from, depending on how much time or energy you have to walk on any given day. Include at least one indoor "route"—an indoor track at a health club, or a local shopping mall—to use during bad weather.

Pollen

Going outside at all during certain times of the year can be a disaster for some of us. One whiff of pollen—especially certain kinds—and we can be in trouble in no time.

*Sometimes TV and radio stations broadcast local pollen counts for your area...but if you want another source for this information you can find it on-line at **www.aaaai.org.***

When you're in or near the pollen season, check to see which pollens you'll be breathing so you can protect yourself.

Finally...after you've been outside for any length of time, always remember to shower to wash away the pollen from your skin and hair. Re-dress in clean clothes.

---

2. **Don't be cheap about the footwear.** The $15 discount house "cheapies" are often poorly made. Your feet and legs need better support. You don't need to spend a lot of money to get better-made walking shoes. Make sure you buy shoes that

"breathe" and are made with fabric (not leather) uppers...
and be sure they support your instep and ankle well.

3. **Get your *walking rhythm* and your *pulse* up.** You'll want to
achieve a rhythm to your stride that is aggressive enough to
encourage proper deep breathing, yet one that you can sus-
tain through most of your walk. You can easily check your
pulse by placing the index and middle finger of your left hand
on your right medial artery—that blue "pencil" line at the
base of the right thumb.

─── *Target Heart-Rate Range* ───

*Below are target heart-rates you'll want to reach if
you'd like to get a good aerobic workout during your
walk (or any other exercise). Achieving your target
rate for at least 30 minutes, 3 times a week, is a very
good thing to do.*

Age	Range
25	117 to 156 beats per minute (20 to 26 beats per 10 seconds)
35	111 to 148 beats per minute (19 to 25 beats per 10 seconds)
45	105 to 140 beats per minute (18 to 23 beats per 10 seconds)
55	99 to 132 beats per minute (17 to 22 beats per 10 seconds)
65	93 to 124 beats per minute (16 to 21 beats per 10 seconds)

4. **Let your mind and spirit relax.** Walking is a great way to release mental, spiritual, and physical stress.

This is an excellent time to pray, unburdening your soul to God. If you prefer, meditate on a *positive affirmation* from Scripture or an inspirational writing.

5. **At the end of your walk, give yourself a good 10- to 15-minute cool-down period.** After elevating your heart-rate, it's not a good idea to sit or lie down immediately. Give your heart-rate a chance to return to normal.

BE CAREFUL ABOUT HEAT AND TOO MUCH SUN

～

Sure, warm weather is very tempting…you just want to be outdoors, putting in a good walk or run.

When you have allergies, your body already has an extra strain on it. Exercising outdoors when it's hot or very sunny can border on self-abuse. The added heat (especially if it's humid) overtaxes your lungs and can trigger respiratory failure. Intense sunlight stimulates histamine production, challenging your skin and mucous membranes. And besides that, you put yourself in danger of heat-stroke, sun-stroke, and worse.

If you really love an outdoor workout, though:

1. Exercise later in the day, after 4 p.m., when the sun's most intense and damaging rays are at a minimum.

2. Listen to local television and radio weather for a report about air-quality and heat-index warnings. *Heed them.*

Strategy #4: Non-Impact Aerobics (NIA)

Non-Impact Aerobics (NIA) offers a great workout experience—minus the pounding intensity of normal aerobics. It's a great way to exercise if you want more than stretching or deep breathing.

NIA is a blend of stretching, fluid motion, *and* proper breathing. The routines are comprised of slower, more graceful movements—and the emphasis on "right form" adds the benefits of muscle toning and elevated respiration and circulation.

NIA was developed by two aerobics instructors, Debbie and Carlos Rosas, who discovered that high-impact aerobics often cause serious injuries for those who jump into those challenging routines without good prior conditioning, and also for people with health conditions.

Note: You can provide your own meditational experience, using Scripture or passages from inspirational readings.

If you cannot find an NIA instructor in your area, you may wish to try Tai Chi—again, seeking a religiously-neutral environment if that's your preference.

Do This

1. Check local community centers, gyms, and health clubs to sign up for NIA classes. Or…

2. Purchase a video-taped version of an NIA workout. These are available in many larger bookstores and through online book and tape sellers.

Strategy #5: Aerobics (Exercise, Dance, or Step)

By adulthood, when we become less physically active, few of us are ready to jump right into a challenging, high-impact aerobic workout. Some cautions apply if your body is challenged by allergies—especially those that affect your breathing.

To Run...to Bike...or to Swim?

Running is one of those physical activities you either come to love or you hate.

If you have allergies, running can be a problem for you. First, there are environmental pollutants—from auto fumes to pollens and other airborne irritants. Second, on days when allergies are acting up, the added stress of pounding the pavement can be extra jarring. Headaches, muscle strains, and greater fatigue will be the result.

Biking takes the heat off your joints and still gives you the fast-paced, out-in-nature workout of a good run. But of course, you're still subject to the elements and airborne pollutants and allergens.

Swimming is a great indoor alternative to running or biking, whether you love the water or just hate the pavement.

People with respiratory allergies generally find they have less trouble with swimming than running. People with skin allergies, however, should be aware that the chemicals used to treat pools—especially public pools—can be harsh on your skin.

Extra Precautions:

- Whenever you are placing a greater strain on your body, be sure you're checked out by a physician, allergist, or a naturopath who is trained to treat allergies. Allow them to assess your overall health condition, and advise you in how to minimize allergic response to outdoor conditions or chemically-treated water.

- If you normally carry some kind of card in your wallet or purse, specifying that you're prone to life-threatening allergic responses (asthma, anaphylactic shock from insect stings, reactions to certain drugs)...remember to wear a bracelet with this information when you run, bike, or swim. If you have a medical emergency, having this information with you could save your life.

Do This

Visit different aerobics classes and decide which kind you'd stick with. If you're a guy and you've always admired the fluid movement of dance…go for it. Try an aerobic dance class—even if you're the only male in it. (Your buddies aren't watching, and why do you care so much what they think anyway?) If you're a woman (or man) who's out-of-shape and you think you'd feel awkward huffing and puffing in the midst of all those more slender people, then consider joining a "slow-start class" designed for people who carry more weight.

In any case…some guidance:

1. **Start slow.** Some aerobics instructors have been at it for years. They can jump right into a fast routine. This is never good for someone who has respiratory allergies. Your lungs need time to open up. You'll be less likely to trigger an exercise-induced episode if you warm up into a full routine.

2. **Stay hydrated.** Remember, you want to keep your electrolytes balanced and avoid drying out your mucous membranes.

3. **Monitor your pulse and respiration throughout your workout.** Use the Target Heart-Rate Chart on page 58.

4. **When you're done, allow yourself a 20- to 30-minute cool-down period.**

Strategy #6: Get Tough—Weights, Martial Arts, Etc.

Allergies have sidelined some of us much of our lives. While other kids were able to play sports, camp, and hike, we sat home snuffling into boxes of tissues. Sometimes allergies have affected our self-esteem.

You may not have a negative view of yourself as a "weakling" or a "wimp," but you may be impaired in your *estimation of what you can do.*

Do you really know your physical limits? Do you know what you're capable of doing physically? Part of achieving "whole-person" health is to test and try yourself. You can experience many overall benefits from putting yourself physically to the test. To do this, you may want to consider serious weight-training, or learning martial art skills, under the guidance of a professional trainer.

If you plan to try one of these more serious forms of exercise you should consult with a healthcare professional in advance. Some trainers will even require it, depending on your age and physical or health condition.

A strenuous program of weight-training or martial arts can increase your body's resistance and return a sense of personal esteem that impairment often erodes. And, of course, a good tough workout also releases health-producing hormones, strengthens immune response, and increases circulation and metabolism.

5

Empowering Your Mind

We know that when we fight allergies our immune system is struggling to fight off an attack that's coming from somewhere *outside* ourselves—from some allergen that's wreaking havoc on our being. But many of us are unaware that *internal* forces can also be at work weakening our immune system, wearing down all our body's defenses.

If we're unaware of these internal forces and don't know how to stop their attacks, we may eat a healthy diet, get good exercise, and take natural supplements...and *still* have breaches in our overall defense.

An "Invisible Enemy"

One of those internal forces—an "invisible enemy" of immune function—comes at us in the form of *mental stress.*

Mental stress becomes invisible to us because we live in a challenging world, and over time we learn how to make room in our lives for more stress than we should. We accommodate all kinds of tensions without any clue as to how that affects our physical person.

Here are several general ways most of us accommodate too much mental stress.

One way is by rationalizing it. We tell ourselves, "Everyone's stressed-out." Or we may think, "If I've got too much on my mind, that means I'm an important person who is needed."

A second way we accommodate mental stress is by ignoring it. We think, "Okay, so I'm confused, overwhelmed, or I forget things easily. So what—that's normal." Or, "I don't want other people to know how often my head is about to explode. So I'll just pretend that doesn't happen to me."

A *third way* is by carrying a vague, unrealistic hope: "Maybe someone else will come and resolve these tensions for me." Or, "Maybe it'll all just go away."

Building Better Mental Habits

Whatever our reasons for ignoring mental stress, it *does* wear on our overall health. Unfortunately, most of us have developed deeply-ingrained mental habits that allow us to accommodate lots of stress for long periods of time. As a result, many of us are what can be called "stress batteries." We store up negative nervous tension in our physical being. We're tense, tight. Our digestion may be off. And often, we don't sleep well.

For allergy sufferers, all these physical effects of stress seriously weaken the immune system. We're less able to resist allergens, and when symptoms kick in they're magnified, and we feel awful. Not only that, our body labors harder and takes longer to fight off the attack.

But we can turn this picture around and learn better mental habits—the kind that prevent stress from crushing us in the first place. We can learn to use simple, tried-and-true techniques to relax and free our stressed-out mind, and at the same time release tension from our body.

Today, healthcare practitioners of various stripes are making fantastic claims about the curative powers of the mind. While there is clearly a basis for those claims, sometimes the claims go a bit far.

No, we don't alter reality, create wealth, cure illness, or change our boss just by adopting the right mental attitude or by the "power" of our thoughts. To have the kind of power on the tip of our tongue that some of today's healers claim we have would be nice—but it's not so. And on the other side, we feel we're to blame for "bringing problems on ourselves" if we have a tendency to be gloomy and speak negatively.

Nonetheless, what goes on inside our head *does* impact our whole being. The mental tension we create or store in our mind sends a sort of "ripple effect" through bone, blood, nerve, and tissue, stressing our whole being. Depending on how we direct the focus and actions of our mind, we can actually add to our illnesses.

Fortunately, there is a positive side. Our mind can play a very important part in boosting our immune function and supporting overall wellness.

What follows is a list of strategies you can use just about any time and anywhere to prevent or overcome mental stress.

Immune-Boosting Strategies for Your Mind

Strategy #1: Get Your Mind Out-of-Gear

If you're looking for the most easy-to-use, "emergency stress-relief technique," this strategy is it. You can use this mentally relaxing technique at home, at work, or even while stuck in traffic. You don't have to "take" anything, and it costs absolutely nothing. Learning this strategy supports the old adage that "sometimes the simple things are the best."

First, stress and intense focus go hand in hand. Find a serious error in your checkbook…your eyes focus in, and all your mental energy is driven into those little pages and columns of numbers. Without realizing it your breathing gets shallow, and your muscles tense up. The minute you find the error—especially if it turns out to be no problem—notice what happens. You look up, heave a sigh of relief, and let your body relax.

When we're stressed by life, the focus of all our energy "zooms in" on a problem. We're engaged in what's called *convergent thinking.* All of our attention and energies are being brought to bear, and our whole being is under stress.

Getting a picture of how your mind focuses may help you understand how to use this strategy. Intense, convergent thinking might appear like the figure in the drawing on page 68. All the energy of your being is focused on a problem. Physically, your adrenaline is pumping, your heart and blood vessels are under pressure, your whole person is being taxed. You feel tense inside, too,

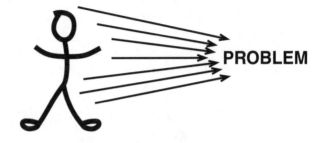

Convergent Thinking

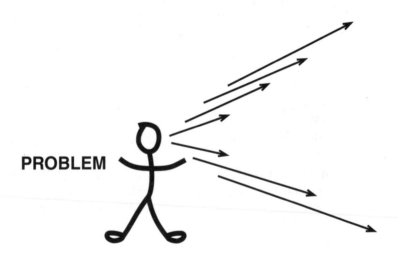

Divergent Thinking

because you're creating a state of inner tension that matches your outer tension.

Fortunately, there is another kind of physical state we can create by learning how to encourage a relaxed or serene focus. We train ourselves to shift to this state when stress is pressing in.

Undoubtedly, you've looked up at a mountain peak or let your eyes wander to the blue horizon or the expanse of sky. What happens?

When we focus "out there," we trigger *divergent thinking*. Our focus broadens as, in a sense, we "step out" of our immediate circumstances…even if they are mentally, emotionally, spiritually, or physically pressured. Our muscles relax, breathing slows and deepens. We experience a sense of restfulness and maybe even total well-being.

Picture divergent thinking as shown in the figure on page 68…and imagine the fluid waves of restfulness you've experienced during a restful wander in nature.

The good news is, you can easily train yourself to make the simple switch from convergent to divergent thinking…and almost instantly relieve stress.

Whether you can walk outside and fix your eyes on clear-blue sky or not, the steps of this strategy are very easy to use.

Do This

1. **Train your eyes on *distance*.** Any horizon or the open sky will do. If you're inside, just let your eyes relax and unfocus. (Your gaze may tend to rise naturally, and you'll be "staring at nothing"—just like when you daydream.)

2. **Breathe in slowly** through the nose and fill your chest. Breathe out slowly through the mouth. Allow your breathing to settle into a slow, deep pattern. (You might want to review the deep breathing strategy described in the previous chapter.)

3. **"Scan" for muscle tension anywhere in your body.** Consciously relax those muscles.

4. **Allow your mind time to rest "out there," beyond yourself.** Very few of us get enough of this "relaxed but alert" mental state. It triggers creativity, inner calm, and physical well-being. This is not by any stretch a "waste of time."

5. **If stressful thoughts come, gently turn them aside.** Set them "behind you" on a "shelf" in your mind, where you can retrieve them and deal with them later. If your muscles begin to tense, release them.

The health benefits of this strategy are almost instant and truly amazing.

Our bodies release *endorphins*—those hormones responsible for giving us a sense of calm and well-being and increasing immune function.

Strategy #2: Lean into Life

Having allergies can become very life-limiting…if you allow it to happen. You stop certain activities you used to like. You don't visit certain friends or family members in their homes. Certain times of the year, you don't even go outdoors very much. Too many allergy sufferers give up more ground than they realize and live limited, restricted lives that are less than full and happy.

Yes, we do need to back up and set limits to protect ourselves from allergens, especially if they make us seriously ill. But we should retreat to a safe zone only until we can figure out how to return to the life we want and restore normal, healthy living as much as possible. Too often, though, we stay in retreat. We may give up and not seek or keep using the help that would actually free us from our symptoms.

One foundational aspect of mental health and a stress-releasing mindset comes from taking the attitude that says *yes* to life. It's this empowering *yes* that allergy sufferers lose, as a swarm of attacking allergens pushes us back and away from the life we want. Adopt a basic attitude that says, "I will make the absolute best of life and not take *no* for an answer. I will find the way to live well, as best I can.

What many of us need is to restore an aggressive, *can-do* sense about life. This subtle but definite change from retreating from our life and our desires, to laying hold of them, restores in us a mindset that leads to well-being. How can we build this mindset?

Do This

1. **Say *yes* to life.** Create a set of affirmations that help you assert yourself toward the goals and desires you have for your life that allergies are now limiting. These may include:

   - **Places you like to go.** Instead of telling yourself, "I can't go there"…try affirming, "I will find a way to enjoy the outdoors again."

   - **Goals you want to achieve.** Instead of saying, "I can never reach that goal" or "do that activity I like"…tell yourself, "I *will* manage my asthma and be involved in strenuous sports again." Or, "I will find a way to overcome my allergy to horses, and learn how to ride."

   - **People you want to spend time with.** Instead of, "I can never go to their house again, so there goes a good friendship," affirm instead, "I will talk about my allergy problems with this friend and find workable alternatives for spending time together."

2. **Picture yourself "leaning into life."** Some of us are motivated by logical thought and by verbalizing our intentions, and the affirmations we create help us stay in the game of life. Others of us are motivated more by feel and intuition…by the creative side of the brain…which is more likely to respond to positive images. If that's you, try fixing an image in your mind whenever allergies cause you to hold back and consider limiting your life—perhaps an image you create for yourself…or one of these:

   - **You are a skier coursing down a mountain slope.** If you ski, you know that leaning back and holding back as you plunge downhill is an almost sure-fire way to fall backwards on your duff. Leaning *into* the slope and skiing it aggressively is what makes the run great.

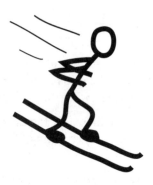

- **You are a runner on a long course.** Maybe you wouldn't be caught dead with "sticks" strapped on your feet, crashing down a mountain. Then picture yourself as a runner with a long, challenging race ahead. If your running motion is all up-and-down, you expend more energy and it's harder to run. Instead, you lean a little forward…into your stride… and momentum carries you forward.

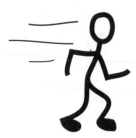

- **You are gliding on roller-blades…or cutting a wave on a surfboard.** Okay, so the strenuous nature of skiing or running is not *you*. Take an image from one of the "smoother" sports. The same leaning motion applies. Picture yourself on an open road, leaning into your glide…or catching the crest of a wave, and tilting forward enough to send your surfboard slicing toward the beach.

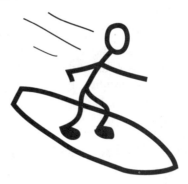

The bottom line of this strategy is that we all need a positively motivated mindset to help us stick with the long road to health and well-being. "Leaning into life" with our personal affirmations and our imagination can help establish a foundational *yes* that keeps us moving toward the answer to even the most life-limiting allergies.

Strategy #3: Assess the Stress…Is It Really Yours?

Sometimes we accumulate mental stress that really isn't ours to carry.

Earlier we talked about people who are "stress batteries," storing tension in their physical being. We can also become "stress batteries" when we pick up mental tension from other people. Here's how it works:

- A spouse announces they have an urgent problem, and they're really not trying to think it through; they're just giving in to anxiety or anger. They storm around until you think it through and figure out how to resolve the issue for them. Or if you can't solve it, you carry the problem around in your head, turning it over and over, trying to think of a solution.

- Someone walks in and unloads a complicated emotional or situational mess. When they leave, *they* feel better…but you feel worse. As before, you carry the worry, anguishing about a solution.

Some of us are in the habit of picking up others' mental stress. We listen because we care about them, but then we carry it off with us, and in so doing we're unkind to ourselves.

Yes, we can and should offer empathy and encouragement where we can. Yes, some people actually do need us to be concerned for them. (Are you sure you know which ones *really* do…and which don't?)

But the fact is, we—and the people in our lives—are actually better off if each of us learns how to shoulder our own personal load. If you have become a "stress battery" because you're absorbing far too many of other people's worries, grouches, gripes, griefs, and complaints…

Do This

1. **Pause and honestly assess every stressful situation someone tries to turn over to you.** Some work is absolutely not yours to do. Solving every problem, being the oracle with an answer to every need and question—this is *not* your work.

2. **Offer the solutions you can, then turn the responsibility back over to the one to whom it really belongs.** We may *think* it's easier to step in and actively solve a problem ourselves. But in the long run we're not doing ourselves or the other person any favors.

   Here's the rule: As often as possible, the person who carries a problem into the room with them needs to be the one who carries it out with them when they go.

3. **Resist the urge to spare other people from the discomfort of struggle and hard work.** We need to let people learn how to wrestle through their conflicts...*without* our constant help and intervention. In this way, others can learn to bear the responsibilities of life, to make mistakes and learn how to succeed, and to make mature decisions.

Allowing others to shoulder the weight of their own challenges has several benefits. It restores *balance* in unbalanced relationships. And of course it eases mental stress that creates undue physical and emotional pressure on us.

Note: *If you genuinely* are *part of the solution to another person's problem, you should joyfully fulfill your role by doing what you can to help. Just be sure that you* are *part of the solution first.*

Strategy #4: "Heal" the Way You Talk to Yourself

Most of us are convinced that our stress is all external, caused by pressuring circumstances and people. It's true, a lot of stress-triggers exist all around us. But...

The truth is, we are the ones responsible for actually making an event or circumstance stressful—or at least adding to it—by the way we respond from within.

One of the biggest contributing factors to mental stress is our *self-talk*.

Self-talk is that interior monologue we carry on all the time, mostly without even realizing it. This running commentary is constantly evaluating, comparing, sizing up, criticizing, judging. Self-talk is based on our deepest beliefs—those "doctrines" and laws of the soul. It's the voice that tells us how to feel and act, and what to say in response to every situation.

This voice is as individual as we are. For that reason, no two people will respond exactly alike to the same circumstance.

Let's say two people have suffered a major career, financial, or health setback.

One person may have a deep faith and a stable family, which offers her a broad base of emotional and spiritual support. Her self-talk may go like this: *"I don't like this. But I can count on God's help. And I know I've got the support of my husband and kids. Bad as this is, I'll get through it somehow."* Her stress level is likely to remain low.

The other guy is the sole supporter of a wife and four kids, and he does not invest as much time in developing a spiritual life. His self-talk may go like this: *"This is a nightmare. I'm furious, and I'm not sure who to be mad at—my boss, the economy, or the whole world. And what if I can't take care of my family? If we have to sell the house, I can't handle that."* His stress level is understandably off the charts, further compromising his health.

Can you see it? It makes a big difference how we interpret events and what we tell ourselves about events. Through our self-talk, we can create mental stress, or we can create calm.

It's well within our power to turn this situation around. And we do that by learning how to tune in to our own inner monologue and learning how to change it.

Here are two ways we can reduce the mental stress generated by our self-talk.

One: Change the way you talk to yourself about life's tough events.

Politicians have made "spin" an art form. They're always telling us how to interpret events. We could actually learn a good mental-health lesson here by learning how to use "spin" the right way. How we *think* about life's hard knocks can actually determine their impact on us more than the events themselves. Consider these two examples:

A serious illness strikes, or we lose someone we love.

- We can pressurize our insides, saying, "This is unfair. I can't live with this pain and tragedy."

- Or we can create a more neutral inner atmosphere with the truth. "Tragedy and loss are part of living. I need to figure out how to adjust my life to this and go on."

A child is in turmoil or lands in serious trouble.

- We can stress out, saying, "I'm a terrible parent" or "My child is a mess."

- Or we can keep the inner pressure down with the truth. "I love my child, even though I don't like what he/she did. But I'll continue to do my best to love, support, and correct him/her, and I understand that I won't always do a perfect job."

Two: Change the way you talk to yourself about yourself.

Some of us spend most of our waking hours launching mental attacks against ourselves. Here are a few examples of negative or destructive self-talk that may be causing you stress.

"What a terrible [parent, worker, partner] I am."

Many of us stress ourselves out with self-accusations and self-punishment. The honest truth is far better for our health: "I make mistakes. I'm human. But there's grace available, and that means I can keep learning and try to do better next time."

"[So and so] is much better at this. I don't have what it takes, and I never will."

Harsh self-evaluations do nothing but increase stress. Comparing ourselves to others who seem capable and happy only grinds us in the dust. Life is about finding out who we are, what we like, and what we're good at. We can say instead, "I might learn a lot about myself if I attempt this. At least I'll find out if I like it and if I'm good at it. If not, I can drop it and go on to something else."

"I need to do this by myself. Asking for help is weak, a sign of incompetence."
"I can't tell anyone about...."

When we're too independent or too secretive, we wind up carrying too many of life's heavy burdens alone. Far better to open ourselves to the give and take of caring, health-giving friendships. We can tell ourselves, "Helping each other and trusting people is what creates friendships. Good friends are a part of what makes life worth living."

As discussed earlier, choose those to help you who can truly be a part of the solution. Don't dump your burdens on someone to simply lighten your load while increasing theirs.

"I knew better. And I still blew it. What a stupid, stupid, stupid person I am."

Such thinking can betray a "legalistic" mindset—one that whispers at a deep level, "Make a mistake and it's all over for you."

"I wanted to say no, but I said yes. What's the matter with me? Why did I let them force me into this?"

This monologue is riddled with blame—towards ourselves *and* towards others. The questions we might better ask are, "Why do I feel guilty saying no?" or "Why do I need to appear so agreeable?" And instead of adding inner pressure to the mix, we can tell ourselves, "I gave in this time. But it's the last time. Next time all I need to tell them is, 'I really can't.' *Period.*"

Strategy #5: Learn to "Flow Through" Your Problems

Ever wonder why allergy symptoms kick in at the worst possible times…when you're already feeling overwhelmed with problems?

Often, when we hit a problem we freeze in our tracks. Mentally, we stress out. Mental stress spreads and becomes physical, emotional, and spiritual stress. Pretty soon we're sick with anxiety. Here come the allergy symptoms.

One cause of this kind of "brain freeze" is our self-talk. We tell ourselves, "I can't solve this one." But *another* cause is this: We haven't trained ourselves in the mental art of "flowing through" a problem…all the way to a solution.

With a little bit of patience, and a few simple steps, we can train ourselves to stop hitting the panic button and learn how to mentally flow our way through difficulties.

But first, *flow thinking* describes the mental state that occurs when we dream, daydream, or get hooked in to our most creative impulses. When we get into the stream of creative thought, we very often come up with great solutions to our problems, and we leave debilitating stress behind.

Do This

1. **Get the picture right.**

   Let's say you run into a major problem. The way through the situation seems blocked by insurmountable obstacles. But you don't *know* that for sure.

   Like most people, your tendency may be to think there's no way *around* your problem and no good way *through* it. A voice inside may be telling you, "Give up. You're done." Instead of listening to a voice that says you're blocked, trapped, stuck…take charge of the situation, like this:

   Imagine you are standing before a vast, rugged mountain range that is blocking your way…

   Sure, it *looks* as if there is no way through. But the truth is, there is no mountain range on earth that humankind has failed to find a way through. So tell the voices of frustration inside your head, "There *is* a way through this problem, and I'm going to do whatever it takes to find the best solution I can."

   Congratulations. Now you've got the right mental attitude. You've just let go of a lot of mental anxiety and redirected that energy into creative thinking. Stress is already easing.

2. **Move closer to the problem. Examine it…and all your possible options closely.**

   Keep the imaginary mountains in your mind's eye. You are an explorer. Every explorer knows that hidden pathways always reveal themselves if you take time and look long enough.

   When faced with a problem or crisis, most of us back off and check out mentally way too soon. Maybe we give in to fear or insecurity. We tell ourselves things like, "I'm not smart enough to figure this out" or, "This is too complicated—way beyond me" or, "Too much work!"

Explorers *keep* searching for new paths through the mountains they face. And in time a way through—however rugged, however much their mettle (and ours) is tested—does open up.

(Explorers also rely on seasoned guides. They don't go it alone; they ask around until they find a guide who knows the particular mountain range they need to cross. In short, seek advice while you keep exploring possible solutions.)

3. **Keep going...one step at a time...through to a solution.**
   Oddly, some of us get midway through solving a problem, and we give up. Sometimes this happens because we don't *want* things to change. Sometimes we just fail to follow through.

   Until you reach a solution:

   Keep in your mind's eye the peaceful, beautiful plains...the wide open way on the other side of the mountain.

   What would the resolution to your problem *look* like? What will it change? Keep going until you reach the solution!

   When the way is long and the challenges many, remind yourself that your goal is not just a problem solved. It's a way to stay free of the mental stress you had before and the way to a better mental state that makes for improved health and well-being.

6

Spiritual Resilience

*S*piritual resilience? What on earth is *that?* You may be thinking, "Whatever it is, how can it help me? I bought this book to learn how to keep these allergies from making my life miserable."

Actually, building spiritual resilience is one of the latest developments in healthcare technology. Latest, I say—though today we're actually rediscovering what ancient healers and people of faith knew centuries ago: The body, mind, and spirit are all interconnected, and each aspect of our being has a powerful effect on the others.

Just think about it. If you suffer a serious injury or illness, one that lays you up for awhile, you begin to suffer mental restlessness and boredom. If you suffer a catastrophic illness, maybe one that's life threatening, you can nose-dive deeper into anger, fear, and depression. The roots of your being—your spirit—are shaken. You can find yourself asking, "Why was I put here?—to go through *this?* And what did I do to *deserve* this misery?"

Studies show that people who sink into deep-level turmoil are far less resilient against illness. In fact, people with little interior resilience can experience physical symptoms that are more intense.

So you see, body, mind, *and spirit* really do interact and affect our health. Often for worse.

Or...for the Better!

If our spirit can bring us *down*, it can also become strong and resilient and *help us* in our fight to overcome the effects of allergies. Our spirit can actually affect our body *for the better*. Positive changes in our spirits will have a positive impact, from deep inside, on our overall health and physical well-being.

For some of us, this is a new idea. But in both the traditional medical community and in its new counterpart—the complementary care community—studies are proving that the state of our spirit can play an absolutely crucial role in helping us to recover health and improve our total quality of life.

The question then is how do we develop a healthy spirit, one that gives us resilience from the inside out?

In this chapter we'll explore spiritual practices that will help strengthen your inner resilience and fight against allergies.

Real Benefits from a Healthy Spirit

We're not going to talk about "tapping into mystical spiritual powers" that are free-floating in the cosmos. And I am not suggesting that the practices introduced below will be the key that manipulates and opens God's heart so that your prayers and wishes are answered with a healing miracle. Instead, these simple spiritual disciplines are known to benefit a person's total being—spirit, mind, and body.

The health benefits I'm speaking of are, in their own way, somewhat miraculous. Developing a simple, daily regimen of these spiritual practices can

- trigger a deep-relaxation response, which in turn

- increases the production of immunity-hormones,

- boosts the production of neurotransmitter chemicals in the brain—those "feel good" endorphins that bring us mental clarity, and

- promotes deep respiration—good breathing—which circulates better-oxygenated blood.

In a moment we'll explore these spiritual practices that can benefit our total well-being. But first, a brief word about these particular practices and where they come from.

Spiritual Disciplines

The practices we'll be looking at often go by another name—*spiritual disciplines.*

For many of us, the term spiritual disciplines is new. But in Christian spirituality, this is a centuries-old term that refers to certain practices well known to strengthen and build health in the innermost being. As herbs are tonics for the body and mind, you could say spiritual disciplines are tonics for the spirit.

For purposes of this book, when I refer to spirit I mean this: *the part of us that holds our deepest values, highest ideals, and strongest beliefs—the "code" we live by.*

As discussed earlier, our spirit—like our body or our mind—can become weak and even sickly. It can be stressed with conflicts and confusion or wracked with the pain of shocks and losses. And if we live in a way that ignores our values, ideals, or beliefs, it can sink into a state of atrophy from disuse. If we continue to live with stress and conflicts, the result can be cynicism, disillusionment, discouragement, or hopelessness at the core level of our being. That is, if we become weak and sick in spirit, we open ourselves to mental and even physical illness.

Many healthcare practitioners have witnessed the phenomenon of someone who is only moderately ill but whose weak spirit causes their health to get worse and worse. Conversely, many people with healthy, strong, vital spirits have conquered some of the worst illnesses—even surviving cancers that should have claimed their lives.

What we need to live well is a resilient spirit, one that is full of a vitality that helps resist every kind of illness. But most of us have never had any training in practices that build such a spirit.

With some practice of the strategies that follow, you can begin to develop deep-level resilience that has a tonic effect on your whole being.

Spiritual Strategies for Health

Strategy #1: Build Strong, Healthy Core Beliefs

Some of our deep-level stress comes from the sense that something—God, life, circumstances, other people—is squeezing or crushing us. But is our stress *really* the result of outside forces pressing in on us?

In truth, a lot of deep-level stress is generated by the *core beliefs* we hold. I'm not referring to religious tenets we can rattle off, but of foundational beliefs we hold to, sometimes so deeply we may not be fully aware we have them. But they're there...often eroding our overall health. But the good news is that if our core beliefs are damaging us—they can be reshaped.

Do This

1. Identify your core beliefs.

   Often, we can sift through our self-talk and pick out our core beliefs. In this strategy we'll be looking for the negative and stressing beliefs that are weakening us from within. Here are three types of core beliefs we may hold:

   One: Beliefs that you are "on your own," without anyone to help you when needed.

   - "It's all up to me. Even though there are people who could help, they won't. I'm on my own."

   - "If I don't do [such and such], then something terrible will happen."

   - "There is absolutely no one else who can do this the right way. I have to do it because if someone else does it, the results won't be as good."

   Essentially, at a deep level you feel isolated with no one you could or would depend on. All the weight of life rests on you. Talk about stress-inducing!

Two: Beliefs about you as a worthwhile human being.

- "Because I have [a certain illness, upbringing, personality, or physical look] I'm not lovable...not even likable. I'm a lesser human being."
- "I'm not like other people. I'm not normal. Because I'm not like other people I'm weird...defective."
- "I did something wrong and it can never be made right again. No one can forgive me. I'm a terrible, terrible person."

Most us question our worth in some measure. The less worthy you believe yourself to be, the more you will carry deep-level stress, which works against your overall well-being.

Three: Beliefs about your relationship to God.

- "[What I'm suffering with] is punishment. God is paying me back for something I did wrong." Or, "God doesn't care about me."
- "This is a trial. I'm being tested to see if I'm worthy. I just have to bear it."
- "Just when I need help, I'm abandoned. I can't even count on God."
- "This illness I have—it's just not fair. God plays favorites, and I'm not one of them."

At your core, you believe God is punishing, careless, indifferent, an abandoner, unfair. All of these can produce self-pity, despair, resentment, or deep anger. These negative stances do not strengthen you...they stress and weaken you from deep within.

2. **Ask God to begin a new chapter in your life...and especially in your spiritual relationship.**

   Many of us have only experienced a superficial relationship with God. We have let life's circumstances tell us what God is like. But life can be tough—and it can be *very* tough for some of us. So when we let life tell us what God is like, God is going to come out looking pretty lame.

You can begin a new relationship with God today. You can do this just by asking,

"God, I want to know who you really are. And I want to have an honest, deep, and true relationship with you. I need to be honest about myself and these negative core beliefs I have. I need to work them out or learn how to let them go. I need to restore peace and well-being deep inside…because I want to live a more healthy life in spirit, mind, and body."

Despite what "nice" and "polite" religious people may tell you, God is not troubled by raw honesty and an invitation to a stronger relationship. All you have to do is to be willing to keep working on and growing in that relationship. So…

3. **Make a commitment to "stay current" with God. Regularly, use the spiritual practices that work for you to help you stay connected.**

Every relationship with God has a unique aspect to it. People with spiritual know-how can tell you how to stay connected to God and keep growing strong and healthy in spirit. But working on the relationship is up to you.

If you've prayed that one-time prayer suggested above, that's not the end of it—it's just the beginning. Growing in spirit is like working out—you can't hit the gym once or twice a week and really expect to make any great gains.

So make it a priority to experiment with the different spiritual practices that follow. Try each one long enough to find out how it can build a healthier spirit in you.

Strategy #2: Spiritual Attitude Adjustment

Most of us experience some measure of deep-level stress because our view of "the way things should be" is way out of alignment with "the way things really are."

Our attitude is, "Things *should* be the way I think they should be. Life should always be fair, good to me, and without serious pain or loss. No one should ever betray, disappoint, or harm me."

Of course life is not the way we believe it *should* be. By adulthood we know that something is seriously wrong with this world. The thing is, we may *know* this in our heads—but many of us have not adjusted our spirits to this fact. In the deepest part of our being we still *want* the world and the people in it to go our way.

This leaves us with a deep-level problem. There is a gap between our head and our spirit…and in that gap a lot of deep-level stress exists. We're left to struggle and wrangle against that tension, and the stress can work against our overall health.

When your back is out of alignment, you may see a chiropractor for a back adjustment. In a similar way, we all need a bit of "spiritual chiropractic care" from time to time. We need a spiritual attitude adjustment.

Do This

Consider these truths. Allow them to give you a deep-level "reality adjustment."

1. **God is God…and we are not.** Many of us have a spiritual problem we don't even recognize. Our system of religious beliefs, or our principled thinking, tells us, "If you live a certain way things will generally go right for you." This means, "If I believe this, and if I do that…life will run the way I think it should run."

   This kind of thinking betrays the desire we all have to control reality. We all want it to go our way. To think we can figure out all the mysteries of the universe and make reality work our way is an attempt to step into the place of God. When the universe and other people don't do things our way, we're left with deep frustration and anger.

   Christian spirituality teaches us the way of humility. Humility simply means knowing our place in the great order of things. We are to remember that God is God and we are not. It's a big mistake to try to step into God's place and think we can run things better by using our human wisdom.

Because we are *not* God, we aren't capable of controlling events or knowing why all things happen the way they do. (Neither are we capable of judging other people because we never know the full story.) Our most productive role in the scheme of things is to face ourselves honestly and to speak up for the truths we have learned by living in the light of the truth.

2. **The world will one day be a safe and a fair place again, but not right now.**

A lot of our stress comes from a deep-running vein of fear. What if our beloved child or spouse is killed, abducted, lost to us? What if we get a terrible illness? Another type of stress comes from the sense that things are not "fair." Rotten people get away with so much. We never get the breaks other people get.

We do well to recognize that this is a world in which unhappy and unfair things happen to many very good people. In fact, they happen to every one of us.

Christianity teaches us that right now the world *is* disordered. On a grand scale, something is deeply out-of-whack here. All our best plans can go bad. All our efforts to protect and safeguard may not prevent tragedy. Too often justice will not prevail. Not right now. Awful things happen to innocent people. For now. Even Jesus Christ acknowledged this when he told the disciples that God "causes his sun to rise on the evil and the good, and sends rain on the righteous and unrighteous."[1]

In short, we do well to adopt an attitude of *acceptance*. Life, for now, is the way it is. We stress ourselves by insisting things are "unfair" and "shouldn't be this way." We create sickness-inducing turmoil by focusing on the terrors and the bad circumstances of life. Things *are* unfair, things are "iffy"—for

---

1. Matthew 5:45.

now. Yes, some people do seem to have it tougher than others. But we do not have to be hung up and over-wrought about "cosmic injustice." *Why* everything happens as it does is not within our capacity to know.

Experiencing this kind of acceptance allows a deep-level calm to fill our spirit—what the scriptures refer to as the "peace of God." And this, inevitably, works to promote our total well-being.

For those of us with strong beliefs, that means learning how to surrender our lives more completely to God. That may mean recognizing we have entrusted certain aspects of our life to God's care—but we never before have entrusted *this* part. It often means recognizing we are too deeply attached to something or someone. We need another "spiritual attitude adjustment."

3. Let people be…just people. Let things be…just things.

Sometimes we're stressed from playing God in other people's lives. We forget that we're just men and women like everyone else…somewhere on a learning and growth curve. We learned by experience…but too often we don't allow others the freedom to have their own learning experiences. We pressure, manipulate, control.

At the same time, we let others take the place of God in our lives. We are terrified that they will leave us, fail us, or fail to be "perfect" in our eyes. We depend on their constant presence and assurance, and sometimes their perfect behavior, in a way that can only be described as idolatry.

We let go of stress and restore peace when we take the attitude that *only God is God*. Only God is perfect, unfailing, ever-present, and never-leaving. People, possessions, positions…things that are *not* God…are only temporary. They are as subject to change, demise, and failure as we are. They are taken out of our lives, and only God knows when and why.

To accept the fact that people and things come and go is to accept the true nature of things. Taking this attitude soon builds in us a sense of healthy *detachment*. We *enjoy* people and things, but we don't *need* them. That's because we are no longer dependent on people or things as the source of our ultimate well-being. Accepting the true nature of people and things, we find ourselves at peace and free to accept them as gifts. We know they are as likely to *go from* us as they were to *come to* us. We become grateful for them. We no longer need to control them, and we free them from bearing the burdens of our demands and disapprovals.

4. **What is lost will one day be restored...what is unfair will one day be made fair.**

Many people experience deep-level stress from living without *hope.*

Christianity teaches us that our peace lies in the hope of a promised new creation. It gives us the attitudes of *expectancy* and *hope.*

Awaiting the time when God will "make all things new"[2] is anything but escapist thinking. It does not teach us to become passive—giving up on the world or ignoring the wrong in it. Rather, it gives us the peace and wise perspective that comes from knowing that all our small efforts now will be rewarded one day when we see all things made new and all wrongs righted.

What I've described throughout this strategy are the attitudes of *acceptance.* Acceptance does not mean giving up and accepting the *status quo.* Instead, we accept the big scheme of things...and then accept that we have a small but important part to play in it.

Whether you have a deep faith or you're just discovering one—allow this practice to help you move from allergy-aggravating stress to an inner, healing calm...and better health.

---

2. Revelation 21:5

SPIRITUAL DETOX

∾

Natural medicine emphasizes "detoxifying" body, mind, and spirit. Certain herbs are used to cleanse the body. Cleansing fasts are sometimes recommended. Here's one way you can detoxify your *spirit*.

- Declare a "fast" on negative core beliefs reflected in negative self-talk. Just for a day, try catching yourself every time your self-talk reveals the belief you are abandoned, being punished, or being judged less worthy by God.

- Watch for the times when you level negative judgments, criticism, blame, and accusations against other people. This will be a real eye-opener…guaranteed! The standard we use to slam other people…will also be the standard we use to judge ourselves.

Most of us need to recognize that the harsh voice we sometimes hear inside, judging, criticizing, and condemning us, is *not* God's voice. Generally, it's our own.

A day of "fasting" from negative self-talk helps to "detoxify" the spirit…and promotes total well-being.

Strategy #3: Confession—Taking Rightful Responsibility

Every one of us lives with a sense that there is a code of conduct we need to live by. A great deal of our deep-level stress is generated by the guilt we feel when we live with the knowledge that we've done wrong.

Sometimes our stress comes from an awareness that we've violated what we consider to be "God's laws." We've lied. Stolen.

Cheated on a spouse. Attempts at rationalizing don't really help. Down deep, something essential in our life's energy is weakened.

At other times, our stress comes from the awareness we've violated our own "code." We live by a sense that we should never let down someone we love—and then we do. And our spirit suffers stress.

Christianity speaks to us about facing our sins and failures. In this age, when feeling guilty is a "bad" thing…it's amazing how many of us are benefiting by owning up to our wrongdoing and learning how to get back on a healthy track!

We all recognize the red light that flashes inside telling us we've done something that violates the code of conduct chiseled into the wall of our spirit. We can respond to that flashing light by ignoring it. Or we can point the finger at everyone else and blame them or point out *their* failures. But these are merely diversionary tactics.

Only when we accept responsibility for our hurtful actions can we turn the picture around. Admitting we're in violation of a code that embodies our spiritual values is our best chance to get ourselves back on the track of wellness in spirit, mind, and body.

When we hide our guilt, we bury it deep inside us. And the negative stress energy it creates eventually promotes sickness. First in spirit…then in body. To accept responsibility is to end the stress that exists between *what we're doing* and *the code we believe in*. It puts us back on the path of balance and well-being. If you want the total health benefits that come from ending this kind of deep-level tension…

Do This

1. Face up to the facts about your behavior. What part of your personal code have you violated?

    The first step *is* the hardest. Who *likes* to face the difficult truth about themselves? It just doesn't come naturally to us.

    What does come naturally is to dodge the truth, to block it from our minds. And when we're pushed, we defend our actions by blaming someone else ("They made me do it") or by rationalizing ("It wasn't *that* bad").

2. **Start a confessional relationship—with a member of the clergy, with a spiritual counselor, or with a spiritual director.**

   Because we all like to duck responsibility, it's a great idea to have someone present to listen when we finally decide to clear the inner atmosphere. And so you'll want to use this strategy of *confession* in the presence of a member of the clergy, a counselor, or a trusted friend.

   It's hard to imagine if you've never done it, but something very good happens when we face another flesh-and-blood person in an atmosphere of sacred trust and admit the worst about ourselves. Why? Because it's easy to kid ourselves into thinking that a harmful violation is "just a momentary slip" when in fact it's evidence of some great need we're trying to meet in an unhealthy and wrong way. It's easy to keep dodging some truth about ourselves that's uncomfortable to own.

3. **Be willing to hear both sides of the truth…and get a more complete picture of yourself.**

   Confession is a way to bring all of our true self out into the open where we can deal with ourselves as we really are. It also helps to bring closure to events that have been *incomplete* because they've been hidden. Those events continue to have power to affect our lives. In that sense, confession is a cap-stone, "capping off" the flow of guilt, shame, and remorse… allowing us to move on.

   Confession can help us in another way.

   Some of us are the *over-responsible* types. We spend way too much time hip-wading around in the murky lower depths of our soul. We seem bent on finding *something* wrong in our words and actions. We are plagued by what the old saints called "a scrupulous conscience."

   Our problem is that we are over-focused on ourselves. But underneath that, we're driven by an unhealthy fear of God— that God is a fault-finder—and not by the enthusiasm that comes from holding a positive, healthy belief in God.

Confession will sometimes turn into an event in which our trusted "confessor" says, "Lighten up. You're too hard on yourself. Shift your focus to what you're doing *right.*"

As we resolve deep-level tensions growing out of guilty conflicts, our spiritual energies are freed up and redirected into maintaining health and well-being.

Strategy #4: Make Amends Where Possible

Pop culture's stress-relief strategies involve learning how to *avoid* tension. Sometimes, however, we have to *face* tension in order to release it. This is true when it comes to wrongs we've done to others.

Do This

When we need to make amends for harm we've caused, nothing says it better than the advice given in Nike's famous ad campaign: *Just do it.*

You'll be amazed at the sense of balance and peace that come when you've made that apology or attempted to right that wrong.

Strategy #5: Empowering Prayer

For many people, prayer is simply "asking for things" or the recitation of someone else's inspiring words—such as the Prayer of St. Francis, the psalms of David, the Lord's Prayer, or the Serenity Prayer. Others have a somewhat more developed prayer life, one that includes offering gratitude or "praises to God."

Here are two very old types of prayer. They offer very practical and powerful health benefits for the whole person, which is why I highly recommend them both.

One: The Prayer of Quiet

Few of us rarely get to experience real quiet—especially inner quiet. The constant head-noise of everyday living has a wearying, even stressing effect.

SPIRIT-BUILDING AFFIRMATIONS

～

In the Psalms, we find a simple, spirit-strengthening technique we can use ourselves.

In many places, the writer addresses his own soul—speaking to it tenderly, lovingly. It's as if he is recognizing that his spirit is an important part of him that carries wounds and can become weak and sick. The spiritual affirmations we find in various scriptures are tools we can use to build spiritual resilience.

Here are just a few health-affirming verses from throughout the Bible, stated here in the form of affirmations you can use.

- **Psalm 3:3-6**—God is the source of health and strength.

- **Jeremiah 30:17**—I can be restored to good health.

- **Romans 8:31**—No matter what trouble or sickness I face, God is not against me. God is *for* me.

- **Third Epistle of John 2**—God listens to my prayers for good health, and He hears them.

Many of us are intimidated by quiet. When it's too quiet we're confronted by fearful or unhappy thoughts and feelings—so we cram our days with noise and action. As a result, we never give ourselves the opportunity to be still and rest at a deep level.

Do This

1. **Find a quiet spot to be alone.** This can be a favorite chair by a window, a rock on a wooded trail, or a park bench. "Quiet" and "alone" are the operative words.

2. **Dedicate the time to God and to whatever sacred work might need to be done in you.** If God is the maker of our

spirits, then God understands what our innermost being needs in a way that we do not. We are turning our will and intentions over to Someone wiser than we are.

3. **Intend on being quiet.** Make it your sole intention just to fully experience the quiet. If you go expecting "lights" to come or to "hear" a divine message, your mind will become active and intent on the wrong thing. And don't look for a "mystical" feeling. You don't need it. Stillness, outside and inside, is the simple goal.

4. **Bring a pad and pen.** When you try *not* to think about life's details they'll clamor for your attention. Quickly write down the grocery item, the appointment, and the thing you must remember to tell someone...then gently turn your focus back to the quiet.

5. **Make a transitional step.** When you try to find inner quiet, you'll notice tiny noises the most. The hum of the refrigerator motor. Wind in the branches. Go ahead and focus on these sounds for a few moments. Eventually, you'll notice the stillness that's there behind all sounds.

6. **Enjoy the quiet inside you.** You may experience a buoyant sense of tranquility and feel more alert, awake, and alive than you've felt before. Or you may experience a peaceful lull...such as you feel before falling asleep. (If you're overtired, like most adults, you may actually need to sleep.) It's not uncommon, in this state, to experience a sense of the sacred, or the holy...and to sense that you are wordlessly in the company of God.

The prayer of quiet restores to us a clarity about our core values...about life, ourselves, those in our care, even things eternal. And at the physical level, you will also experience deep relaxation.

Two: Contemplation

Contemplation may sound otherworldly. But every day, lovers practice contemplation. It's what we do when we fix the one we love in our mind's eye and dwell on all their best qualities. In a sense, we "take them into us" and let the fact that they are "ours" lift our spirit.

Most often, we let ourselves become over-focused on the gritty and the negative in life. Or on all these wonderful modern conveniences we own that keep breaking down. Or on relationships we depend on and which stress and disappoint us.

The media doesn't do much to boost our spirits. From our inner being we sense a "flatness," even emptiness. A "who cares?" attitude takes over.

We need the restorative spiritual lift contemplation gives.

Do This

Begin as you would with the Prayer of Quiet, in a secluded place. Then:

1. **Focus on something that inspires in you a sense of beauty, orderliness, gratitude, wonder, joy, the holy, love.** This might be an object from nature or a special passage from the scriptures...or some aspect of God—say, God's creativity, gentle care, strength, purity, loyalty to us, or love. These qualities have another name: *graces.*

2. **You might want to start by focusing on the grace of *love*.** We are loved, at all times...whether our immediate circumstances are easy or difficult. And amid all the mixed circumstances of life, we have much to be grateful for...much that would show us we are loved if we will but take the time to look for all its subtle evidences.

3. **Focus on the evidences of love *in your life*.** It's one thing to meditate on some high, disembodied, spiritual concept like love. It's another thing to *notice* love...or the benevolent gifts of God in the everyday stuff of our lives. We can notice benevolence...in the simple loyalty and everyday care of a friend or spouse...in the companionship of a beloved pet...in the traits, gifts, and talents we were given to help us through life...even in the gift of life itself.

Note: Contemplation will have the wonderful effect of helping you sense, not what you "should" be focusing on, but on what you need. (This is not about learning to "count your bless-ings.") Your own spirit will tell you what you're longing for in your everyday life.

For instance, you may find yourself contemplating not on love but on the graceful orderliness of nature. As this grand sense of order inspires you, you may realize your spirit is crying out for beauty...and that your life and relationships are too chaotic.

And so contemplation—which we in the west have shunned as "too mystical"—actually leads us to a very prac-tical next step (which is one of the main points of doing it):

4. **Consider what adjustments you might make in your everyday life, based on the particular spiritual grace that has given you the lift you needed.** There is not much point, really, in having a few lovely moments thinking about a spiritual grace like love or order or truthfulness...if it stops there. We have just experienced a profound connection with our deepest values...the qualities our spirit prizes and hungers for most. Now our task is to make a space in our everyday world for the spiritual reality we prize.

   Ask yourself: How can I give and receive more love? What part of my life needs more order? In what relationships do I want more truthfulness?

Try both these kinds of prayer, and you'll quickly experience the "tonic" benefit they have on spirit, mind, and body.

Clear Health Benefits

This chapter has had a necessarily spiritual tone to it. And so I want to close by focusing directly on the overall health benefits spiritual practices offer—especially the ones that benefit allergy suf-ferers.

1. When we release guilt and shame...when we relieve anxiety and isolation...we release the deep-level stress we've carried.

We trigger the deep-relaxation response, which is necessary to release hormones that strengthen immune function.

2. As stress goes, deep breathing also improves. We increase cardiovascular functioning and the circulation of better-oxygenated blood.

3. Finally, we are more connected to other people and to life itself...improving that other essential combatant we need for good health—*the will to be well!*

Other books by David Hazard in the Healthy Body, Healthy Soul Series

~

Reducing Stress
Simple techniques to reduce stress—from relaxation to herbal teas.

Breaking Free from Depression
Life is good. Don't lose any more time to crippling depression.

Building Cancer Resistance
Simple ways to boost your immune system's resistance to cancer.

Relieving Headaches and Migraines
When taking an aspirin isn't enough—here's the next step.

Controlling PMS
Busy women don't have time to be distracted by the mood swings and discomfort of their menstrual cycle. Here are simple, natural ways any woman can use to minimize the effects of PMS and keep her energy level high.

The New Nature Institute

~

The *New Nature Institute* was founded in 1999 for the purpose of exploring the connection between personal health and wellness and spirituality with the Hebrew-Christian tradition as its spiritual foundation.

Drawing upon this tradition, the Institute supports the belief that humankind is created in the image of God. We are each body, mind, and spirit, and so intricately connected that each aspect of our being affects the other. If one aspect suffers our whole being suffers; if all aspects are being supported we will enjoy a greater sense of well-being.

For this reason, the Institute engages in ongoing research in order to provide up-to-date information that supports a "whole-person" approach to wellness. Most especially, research is focused on the natural approaches to wellness that support health and vitality in the body, the mind, and the spirit.

Healthy Body, Healthy Soul is a series of books intended to complement treatment plans provided by healthcare professionals. They are not meant to be used in place of professional consultations and/or treatment plans.

Along with creating written materials, the New Nature Institute also presents seminars, workshops, and retreats on a range of topics relating to spirituality and wellness. These can be tailored for corporate, spiritual community, or general community settings.

For information contact:

The New Nature Institute
Attn. David Hazard
P.O. Box 568
Round Hill, Virginia 20142
(540) 338-7032
Exangelos@aol.com